COMPELLED by LOVE

THE STORY OF
RUN 4 HEAVEN'S GATE

*How runners and walkers are changing
the lives of children in India...*

Compelled by Love: The Story of Run 4 Heaven's Gate
How Runners and Walkers are Changing the Lives of Children in India

By Amy Hoppock with Dottie Bledsoe, Lauren Phillips, and Maryanna Young

This project was coordinated in collaboration with Calvary Chapel Boise, Send Hope, and Calvary Chapel Trust.

© 2015 by Dottie Bledsoe, Amy Hoppock, Lauren Phillips, and Maryanna Young

All rights reserved. Use of any part of this publication, whether reproduced, transmitted in any form or by any means, electronic, mechanical, photocopying, recording, or otherwise, or stored in a retrieval system, without the prior consent of the publisher, is an infringement of copyright law and is forbidden.

Disclaimer: While the publisher and author have used their best efforts in preparing this book, they make no representations or warranties with respect to the accuracy or completeness of the contents of this book and specifically disclaim any implied warranties of merchantability or fitness for a particular purpose. The advice and strategies contained herein may not be suitable for your situation and you should consult a professional where appropriate. Neither the publisher nor author shall be liable for any loss or profit or any other commercial damages, including but not limited to, special incidental, consequential, or other damages. Consult your healthcare provider before beginning any vigorous exercise program. The information provided herein is in no way intended as a substitute for counseling or other forms of professional guidance. While all the stories reflect true and accurate information, the names of the children have been changed to protect their privacy.

ISBN: 978-1-612061-10-8

Cover Concept by: Doug McFerrin
Interior Design and Cover Layout by: Fusion Creative Works, www.fusioncw.com
Photography by: Full Cup Photography
Project Manager: Hannah Cross

Published by

ALOHA
PUBLISHING

AlohaPublishing.com

First Printing
Printed in Canada

COMPELLED BY LOVE

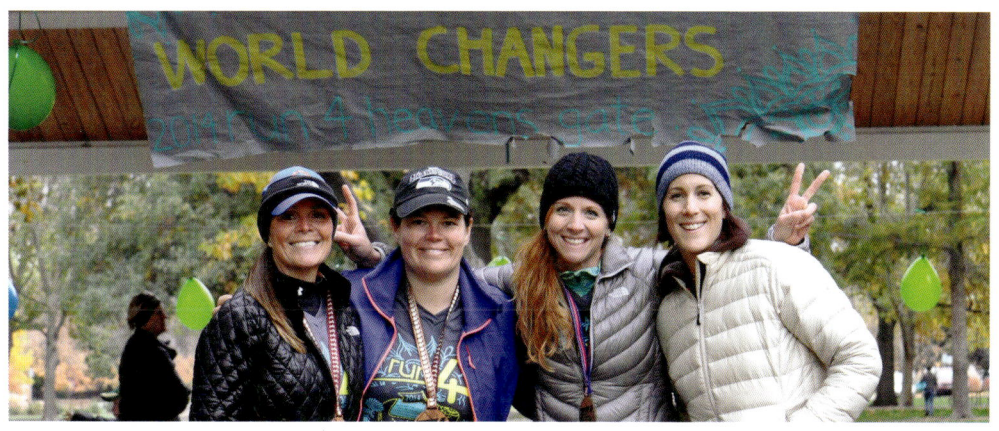

TeriAnn Lukehart, Lindsey Lonseth, Dottie, and Ylonda Hays

When Run 4 Heavens Gate started in 2008, I had no idea what God had in store for me and so many others whose lives have been touched by the simple act of running. It's amazing to see what happens when people come together with a common goal and each does their part. It's a beautiful thing.

These children are real. They are unique and special, created for a purpose, just like you and me. I pray that by reading their stories, their little lives will impact yours and that you will tell others… and their memories will live on.

My hope is that this book will be an inspiration to you. As you read the stories of the runners and the beautiful children in India, you will identify with their joys and sorrows, and be inspired to go out and live your unique life to the fullest. I pray that you will be motivated to use your gifts to make a difference in the lives of others and that you will see the beautiful story God is writing through the lives of ordinary, everyday people – people just like you.

I hope you are inspired to discover the world changer in you.

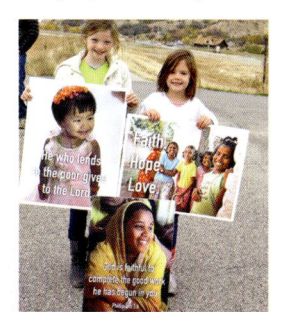

Dottie

To every Run 4 Heaven's Gate runner and walker, we dedicate *Compelled by Love* to you.

To every Heaven's Gate child, we are *Compelled by Love* to run for you. We love you. Your story matters.

To our supporters, sponsors, and encouragers, your generosity and love is our fuel.

COMPELLED BY LOVE

WHAT FOLLOWS IN THE PAGES OF THIS SMALL BOOK IS A STORY OF FAITH, COURAGE, BOLDNESS, AND FEET...

Feet of ordinary people who put on sturdy shoes to run or walk hundreds of miles during training for Run 4 Heaven's Gate: 52.4 miles of love. Their completion of four half marathon races in 30 days supports orphan children suffering with HIV/AIDS in India. They *intentionally* subject themselves to shin splints, achilles injuries, IT band pain, blisters, and lost toe nails (injuries common to distance runners) to bring love, nutrition, and education to suffering children in India.

Feet of men and women in India who willingly walk into some of the filthiest, most disease ridden streets imaginable over animal and human waste to serve a child or families in desperate need. They dig babies out of trash heaps, rescue abandoned children at train stations, and give lost children a place to live and grow in love. They walk through stigma and scorn that surrounds people with AIDS to embrace them with love and vital nutritional support that is literally changing lives, one family at a time.

Feet of leaders who courageously follow God's call. Pastor Guna followed God to Idaho and back to the slums of India. Pastor Bob followed God to India and back to Boise sharing the need, partnership, and support.

God has done and continues to do amazing things through the bearers of ordinary feet: people who choose to step out in faith. Our hope is that you will be challenged to use your feet to change the world as you read about beautiful feet in this book.

COMPELLED BY LOVE

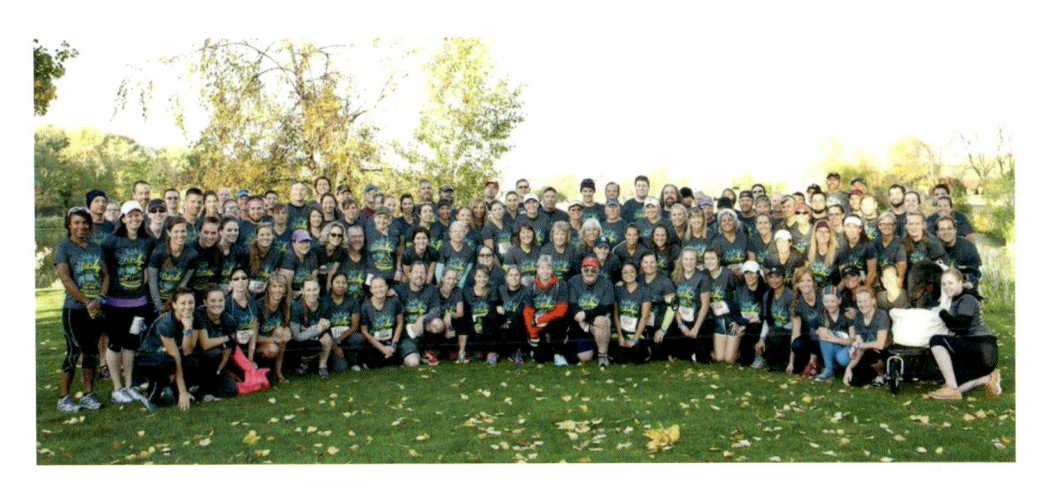

"How beautiful are the feet of those who bring good news!"
– Romans 10:15 NRSV

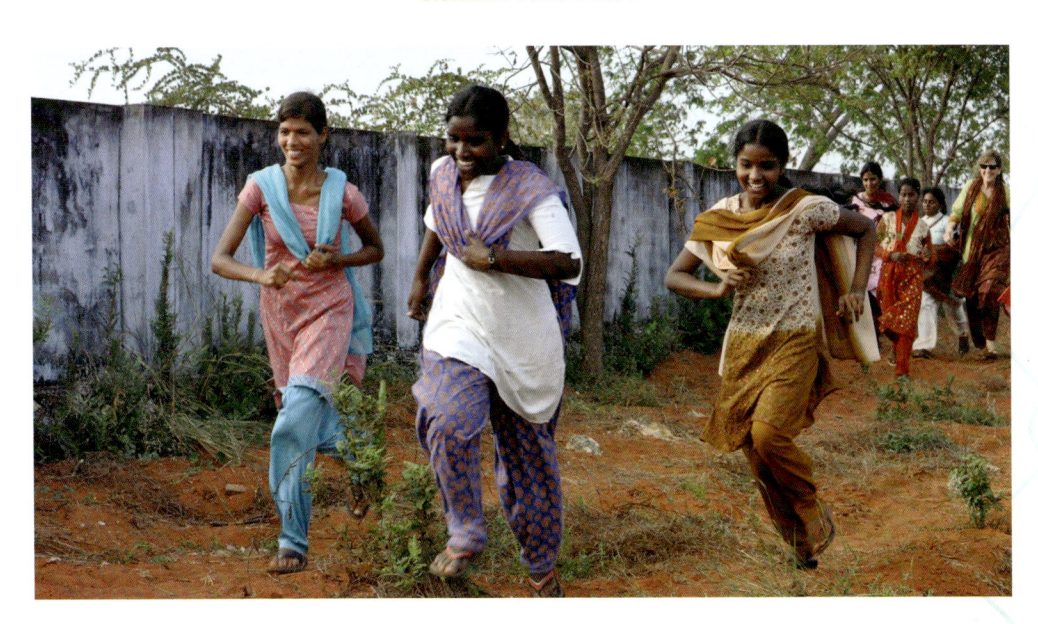

COMPELLED BY LOVE

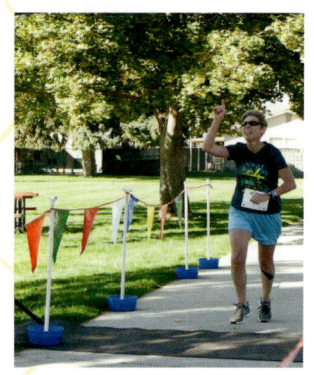

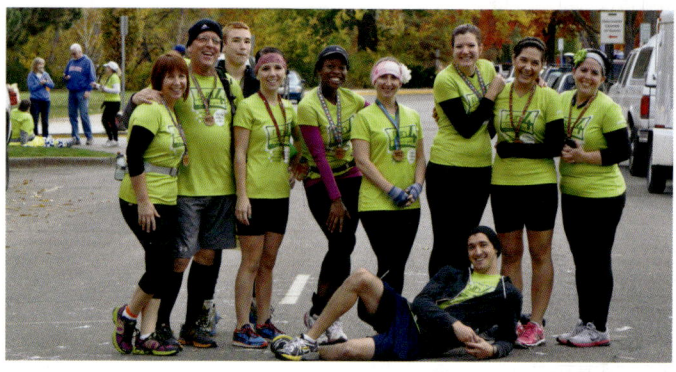

Runner Maryanna Young completing her first of four R4HG races

Mountain Home R4HG Team, 2013

COMPELLED BY LOVE

It's an unlikely story. Four half marathon races completed in four weeks' time, accomplished runners, and complete beginners (walkers too!) challenge themselves with a difficult physical accomplishment to in turn, change the lives of children and families with HIV/AIDS in India. Thousands of miles have been logged, countless pairs of shoes worn out, and lives have been changed.

It's easy to think the runners in the United States–men and women living in a land of abundance–are the givers. However, the lines quickly blur. As stories unfold, it's hard to tell which direction hope is flowing, whether from the children in India or from the runners in Idaho. Though most runners and children have never met, there is a tangible companionship that exists across the ocean.

Run 4 Heaven's Gate is a series of four half marathons completed in four weeks (13.1 miles x 4 weeks = 52.4 miles). Although the results of this effort are significant, the cause's beginning was meager and fueled simply by prayer, teamwork, and passion. In 2014, the seventh year of R4HG, 150 runners and walkers raised more than $160,000. Since the beginning, the "each person can change the world" mindset propelling this effort has provided about a half million dollars of resources to the children of India living with HIV/AIDS. It all began with a desperate mother's request of help for her daughter with HIV, two pastors who didn't listen to common sense, and an American mom who believed running could somehow play a part in changing a child's life.

COMPELLED BY LOVE

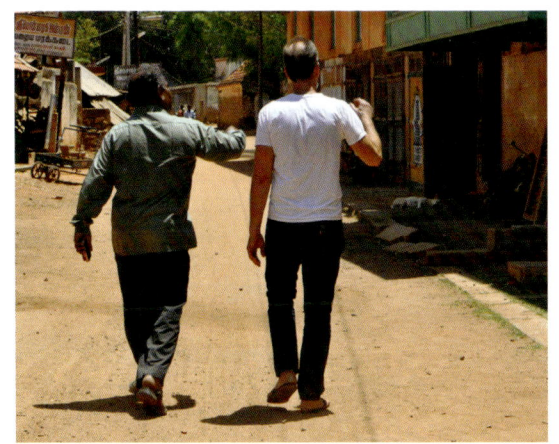

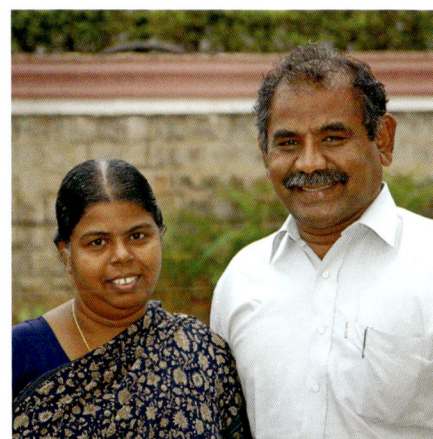

Pastors Bob and Guna walking together in southern India, 2013

Victoria and Guna

Over 25 years ago, Bob Caldwell, pastor of Calvary Chapel Boise, journeyed to India on a vision trip, hoping to uncover how his heart's longing to be involved in India could be realized. At the very same time, Lamech Gunasekaran (Guna), an Indian businessman, was in Idaho working to develop business contacts for his silk import business. Guna and his wife lived a comfortable life in Bangalore, India; he worked as an overseer in the orphanage system that he had grown up in. Wanting more for their family, they sold the only thing of real value, a slender silver necklace that was his wife Victoria's wedding necklace (similar to a wedding ring). The sale of the necklace gave Guna the money for a one-way ticket to America, where he was optimistic he would make money. Garden Valley, Idaho was his unlikely destination.

Guna quickly realized that life in America was not easy and he faced unexpected challenges in Idaho. While delivering flowers to Albertson's, he spotted a small church nearby. Discouraged and looking for some help and hope, he went in. "That day I was upset in my life, no spiritual guidance was given by anyone in America, so when I saw the church I entered into the church just to spend time and pray," Guna recalled. The assistant pastor, surprised at the irony of seeing an Indian man while their lead pastor was in India, welcomed Guna and listened to his story. The church members invited him to stay until Pastor Bob returned from India.

Bob and Cathy Caldwell praying for a young orphan girl, 2002

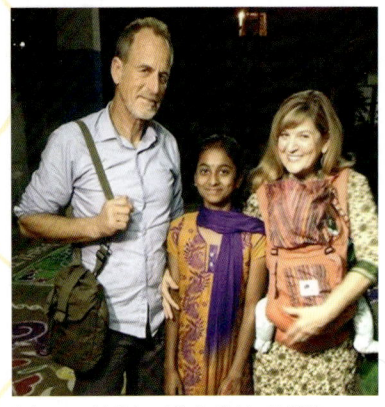

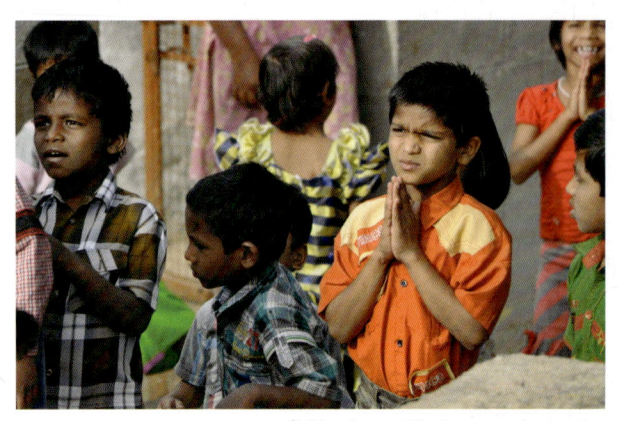

Anjamma with Bob and Cathy Caldwell, 2014

Children in one of the homes praying together

While in Bangalore, Bob, searching for direction, didn't know that God was already working to answer his prayer in his own small church back in Boise.

When Bob returned from India, Guna spent three months living with the Caldwell family receiving intense discipleship. Guna eventually returned to India and went back to his old job, but with a fresh passion to reach out to the local people living in a nearby slum. He started visiting the home of a coworker who lived in the slum, getting to know the family and sharing about the hope found in Jesus.

The ministry grew organically and, led by the Holy Spirit, people came to know Jesus. Guna and his wife Victoria made the courageous, bold, and loving decision to move into the slum with the people they had come to love. People started bringing abandoned children to them, which eventually led to starting their first orphanage. As Bob and Guna were obedient with each new step, more opportunities to love and serve forgotten, broken, and lonely people presented themselves. And so Calvary Chapel Trust was born. In 2007, Bob and Guna, who had built a reputation of kindness and willingness to help, were in an Indian train station when a woman and young girl approached the two men. The desperate mother implored them, "My husband is dead; he died of AIDS. My daughter Anjamma and I both have AIDS. I need your help."

COMPELLED BY LOVE

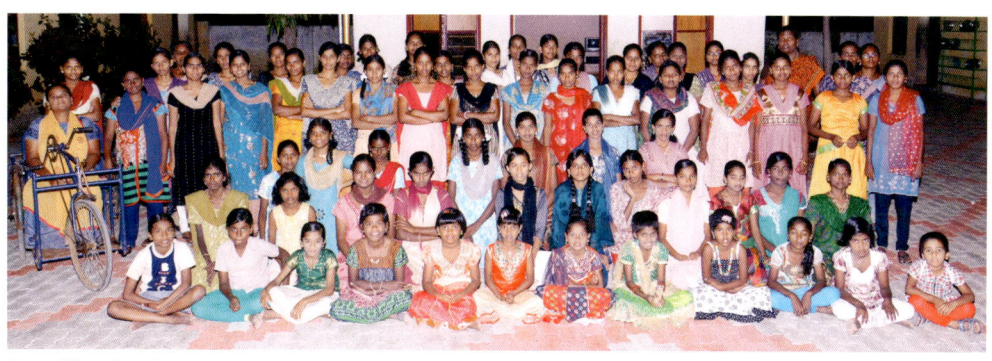

Home of Hope, Anandapurum

Another divine appointment was unfolding for the ministry unbeknownst to Bob and Guna at that pivotal moment. "My first thought was that we cannot agree to help with HIV positive people. It's too big of a problem and too confusing. My next thoughts were how do you bring the gospel into this and not make it a big social program. I have all of this going on in my head and then I realize: all that is ridiculous, who really cares? What matters is these ladies need help and we'll do whatever we can to help them. It changed what we did and now we have 12 different orphanages for children with AIDS," Bob recalls.

Run 4 Heaven's Gate participants run to support Calvary Chapel Trust Homes of Hope orphanages and the community wide HIV/AIDS prevention and care work that has resulted. Calvary Chapel Trust is the Indian partner of Send Hope, the North American arm of the organization based in Boise, Idaho.

The expertise and leadership Calvary Chapel Trust through Send Hope has developed serving those with HIV/AIDS has opened many unexpected doors to help individuals and families suffering with this terrible disease. What seemed like something outside of the scope of the ministry has turned out to be a key that has opened many doors for the growth and expansion of the ministry.

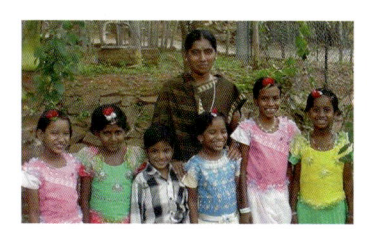

Some of the first HIV/AIDS children to live in the Home of Hope, including Anjamma, 2008

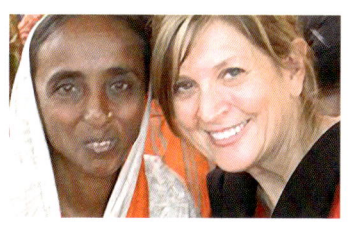

Cathy Caldwell with Anjamma's mother, 2007

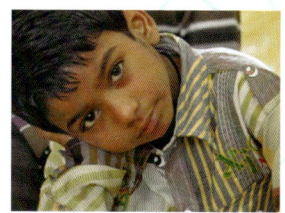

Boy with HIV/AIDS living in Varanasi

COMPELLED BY LOVE

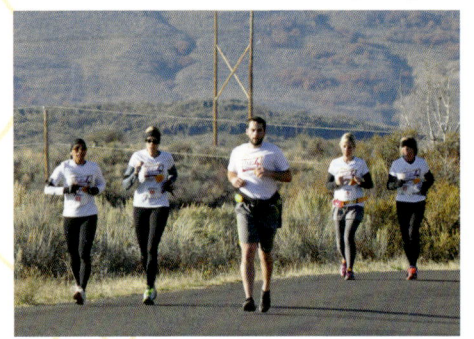

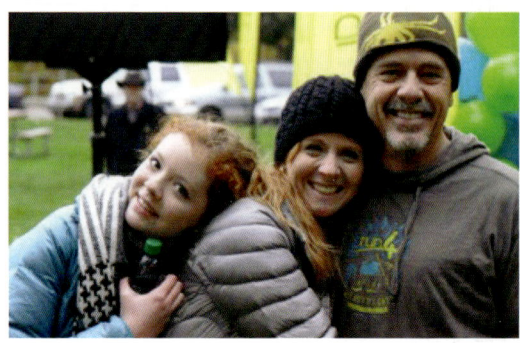

R4HG runners in 2013 at the Rush Creek Stampede Half Marathon, Cambridge, Idaho

Arlie, Dottie, and Steve Bledsoe at R4HG Half Marathon, 2014

If there is a theme that runs through the Calvary Chapel Trust's history, it is ordinary people refusing to be stopped by obstacles. Dottie Bledsoe accepted a challenge she felt in her heart to find a small way to make an impact on behalf of the children in India after her husband Steve returned from a trip where he met the children and saw the need first hand. Those who know Steve know his huge love for children. To say the kids in India captured his heart is an understatement.

"Little things become big with God." – Dottie Bledsoe

Running had been transformational in Dottie's life, so it was natural for her to look to running as a way to begin something extraordinary. "I never felt confident in anything athletic as a teen. Discovering running as an adult was a big thing in my life." She started running on her 21st birthday, the same day she stopped smoking.

As she began to take steps towards a healthier lifestyle, she still felt so much emptiness and knew something was missing. "Then, to put it simply, I found Jesus. As my relationship with Him grew, I found myself finally ready to make changes in my life after years of rebellion and pain. The direction of my life changed when I let Jesus take over, and I am forever grateful."

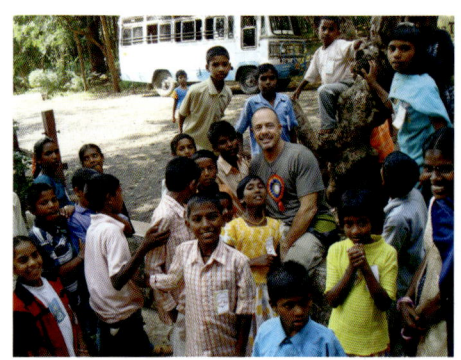

Steve in India, 2007

COMPELLED BY LOVE

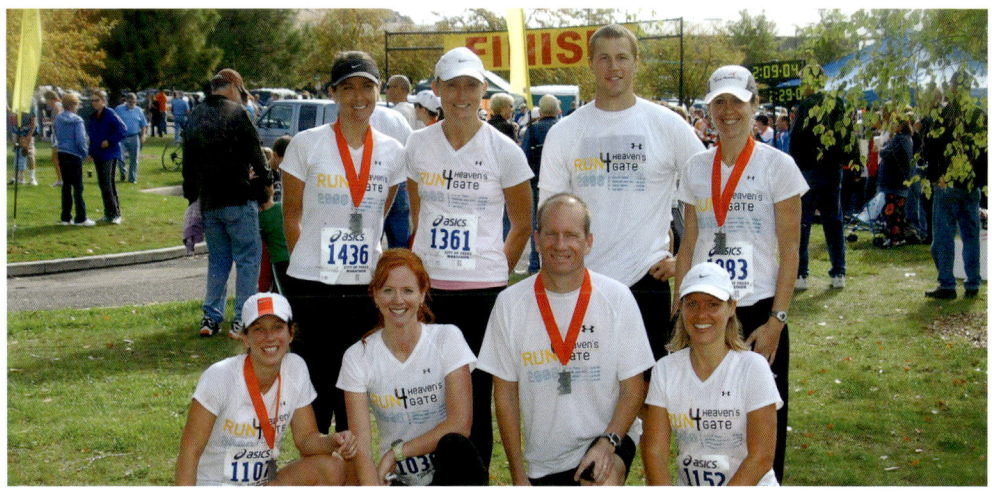

The original R4HG team, 2008
Top Row from Left: Mer Versaggi, Angie Thorenson, Tyler Moyer, Alyssa Daley
Bottom Row from Left: Melinda Eldfrick, Dottie Bledsoe, Mike Slaughter, Amy Haugen

After Steve returned, they started brainstorming about ways they could help. Knowing that the ministry had just started taking in children with AIDS, they wanted to find a way to help raise money specifically for children with HIV/AIDS. While on a road trip with his family, Steve, a business owner and outside of the box kind of guy, had an idea. "What about four races in four weeks?"

"I loved it," Dottie recalls, "And I just knew that it would work." Over the next few weeks, while on her regular morning runs, she talked about it with her girlfriends and the idea began looking more like a reality. Shortly thereafter, she called Lauren Phillips, administrator of Send Hope at Calvary Chapel, and told her of their idea.

A simple announcement was put in the Boise church's bulletin; Dottie and Lauren waited to see what would happen. Dottie and seven other runners ran the first Run 4 Heaven's Gate race season in 2008. "We all had the same purpose and heart. Together we raised $13,000! I was amazed!"

Five years after the first R4HG season, Dottie had the opportunity to travel to India and see the impact Run 4 Heaven's Gate was making. "I was really excited to see what was being done and how far the money went. I came home overwhelmed. The need was so huge and seemed never ending."

COMPELLED BY LOVE

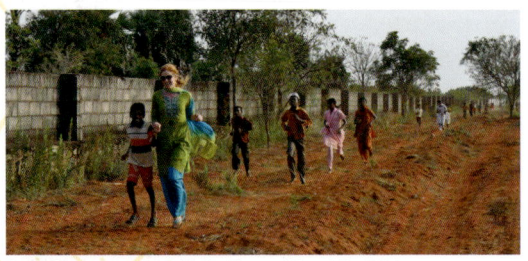

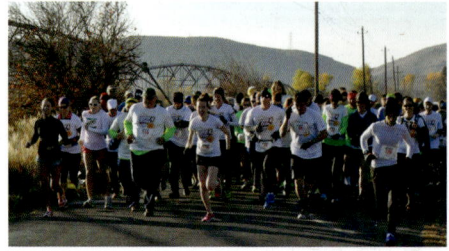

Dottie Bledsoe running with the Home of Hope kids, 2011

Start line of Rush Creek Stampede Half Marathon, 2012

During that trip, Dottie had a chance to run a two-mile loop around one of the homes with children who lived there. "It was a surreal moment. All of the kids ran, and even children sick with AIDS walked the course. For me, that simple run was the culmination of my entire journey starting Run 4 Heaven's Gate. It was awesome to be there with kids and to see first hand how we (the team and the children) are all knit together. It was after that run that the children began to understand the sacrifice the runners make for them. They now understand how much we all love them and they know that they are worth the sacrifice."

Dottie has been able to merge two life passions–running and orphaned children in India–and the impact of following her passion has touched countless lives in both Boise and India. People in Boise who never thought of themselves as runners have learned the joy that comes from putting on running shoes and logging mileage alone or with others. Trials have been overcome, prayers have been answered, and lonely people have found friendships. Children in India have found hope, love, family, and Jesus. Medical care has been given, food has been shared, suffering has been lessened.

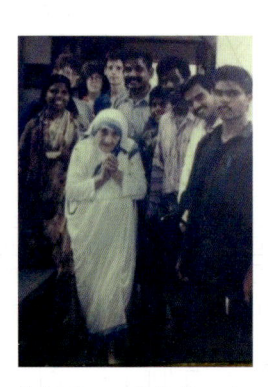

Mother Teresa with the Gunasekarans, 1990s

I never look at the masses as my responsibility; I look at the individual. I can only love one person at a time – just one, one, one. So you begin. I began – I picked up one person. Maybe if I didn't pick up that one person, I wouldn't have picked up forty-two thousand... The same thing goes for you, the same thing in your family, the same thing in your church, your community. Just begin – one, one, one.

– Mother Teresa

COMPELLED BY LOVE

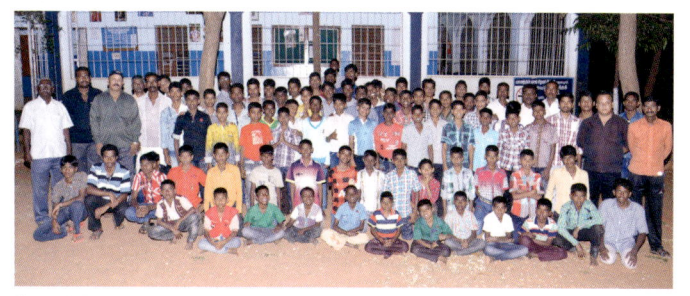

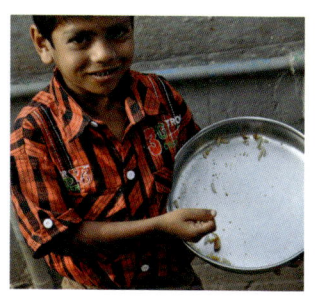

Nazareth Boys Home, Thailapuram

Calvary Chapel Trust welcomes all children and their extended families regardless of their religion. Homes of Hope provide a loving home, complete with medical care, education, and the love of Jesus, to more than 500 orphans in India. Currently close to half of the children living in the Homes of Hope have tested positive for HIV/AIDS. In most cases, these children contracted HIV in utero and have lived with HIV all their lives. Other children have become infected by unsanitary needles used on multiple patients in make-shift doctor's offices in rural India. The HIV virus is spread via bodily fluids and transmitted "vertically" from mother to child.

Up until the early 1990s, AIDS was taboo in India. Public health education was lacking, which fueled the spread of HIV. Additionally, human trafficking, child marriage, and marital infidelity contribute to climbing HIV rates. After acquiring HIV, if left untreated, it often develops into AIDS, a disease which weakens the immune system, ultimately leading to death.

Calvary Chapel Trust's caregivers have become experts in caring for children with HIV, allowing more and more children to be taken in. Special relationships with local hospitals and government programs have been developed. Through love, care, and knowledge refined over time, children in the Homes of Hope are living longer lives than is typically expected for patients of HIV/AIDS in India.

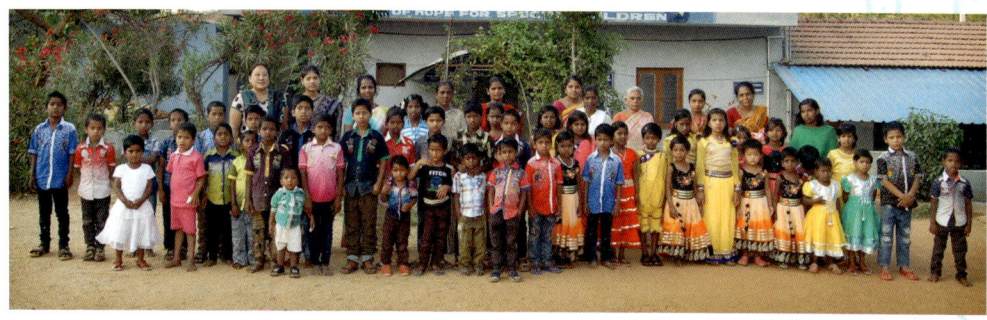

Boys and Girls Home of Hope, Bangalore

COMPELLED BY LOVE

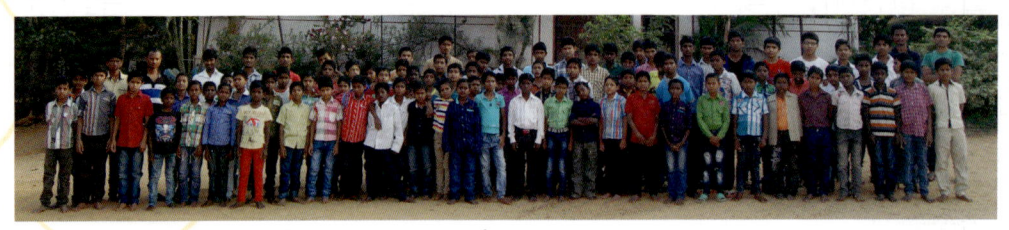

Boys Home of Hope, Bangalore

Calvary Chapel Trust workers not only provide food, medicine, and advocacy for these children, but bring education and the love of God into impoverished slums and forgotten rural areas throughout India. One common way of using their expertise with HIV/AIDS is holding medical testing days. Testing for malaria, TB, and HIV/AIDS is offered and confidentiality is ensured. Within these primarily Hindu communities, there is great stigma attached to those who test positive for HIV/AIDS. One who has HIV/AIDS may be forced to quit working and even pushed out of the community. It is not uncommon for a husband to abandon his family in order that they may continue to live in their village without the shame associated with the disease.

If someone tests positive for HIV/AIDS, the orphanage workers help them gain access to government treatment programs and provide monthly food bags. The role of proper and adequate nutrition for someone with HIV/AIDS provides improved quality of life.

Calvary Chapel Trust has also established more than 100 churches across India, many of which are working in the most difficult and desperate slums and rural areas of India ravaged by extreme poverty.

The impact of those who support Run 4 Heaven's Gate starts with the children and reaches far beyond.

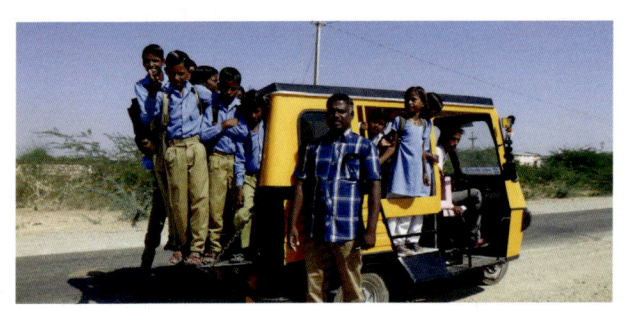

Home of Hope "school bus" in Gujarat

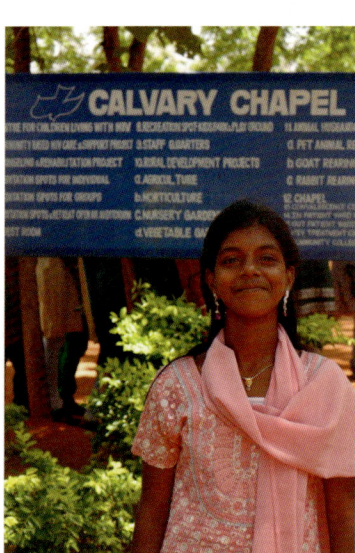

COMPELLED BY LOVE

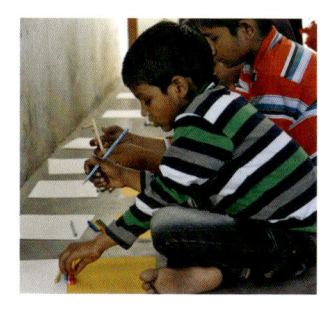

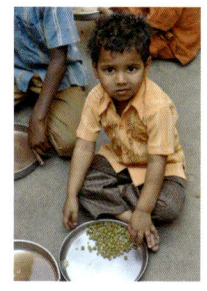

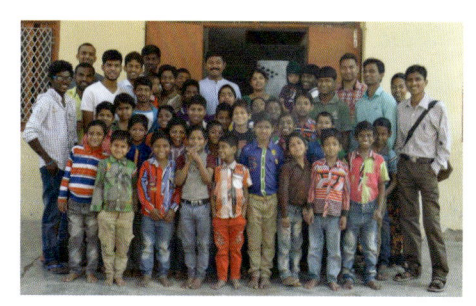

Home of Hope, Varanasi

Currently there are 12 orphanages under the Home of Hope banner located in the six Indian states of Karnataka, Tamil Nadu, Gujarat, Uttar Pradesh, Odisha, and Manipur. At one of the homes in Tamil Nadu, a K-5 Christian, English-medium school for the children in the orphanage and for children from the surrounding villages, regardless of caste or religious background, is run and staffed. Each home is equipped with staff and supplies to care for HIV infected children.

Annual cost of care for a child: $840 (additional for medical care, hospital stays, etc.)

Home of Hope staff: 83 (includes drivers, gardeners, care staff. Many of the assistant drivers, gardeners, gate keepers, etc. are former home children.)

Home	Location	# of Children
Home of Hope Boys and Girls	Bangalore, Karnataka	56
Home of Hope Boys	Bangalore, Karnataka	122
Home of Hope Senior Boys	Bangalore, Karnataka	7
Home of Hope Girls	Bangalore, Karnataka	89
Home of Hope Girls	Anandapuram, Tamil Nadu	76
Home of Hope Boys	Thailapuram, Tamil Nadu	75
Home of Hope Boys and Girls	Nachikuppam, Tamil Nadu	61
Home of Hope Boys	Ranchi, Odisha	10
Home of Hope Boys	Manipur	19
Home of Hope Boys	Varanasi, Uttar Pradesh	29
Home of Hope Girls	Varanasi, Uttar Pradesh	Under Construction 2015
Home of Hope Boys	Gujarat	2
	TOTAL	546

COMPELLED BY LOVE

HIV/AIDS CARE & NUTRITION

HOME OF HOPE LOCATIONS

1 – Special Children
Bangalore, Karnataka 56

2 – Boys
Bangalore, Karnataka 122

3 – Senior Boys
Bangalore, Karnataka 7

4 – Girls
Bangalore, Karnataka 89

5 – Girls
Anandapuram, Tamil Nadu 76

6 – Boys
Thailapuram, Tamil Nadu 75

7 – Children
Nachikuppam, Tamil Nadu 61

8 – Boys
Ranchi, Odisha 10

9 – Boys
Manipur 19

10 – Boys
Varanasi, Uttar Pradesh 29

11 – Girls
Varanasi, Uttar Pradesh
(under construction)

12 – Boys
Gujarat 2

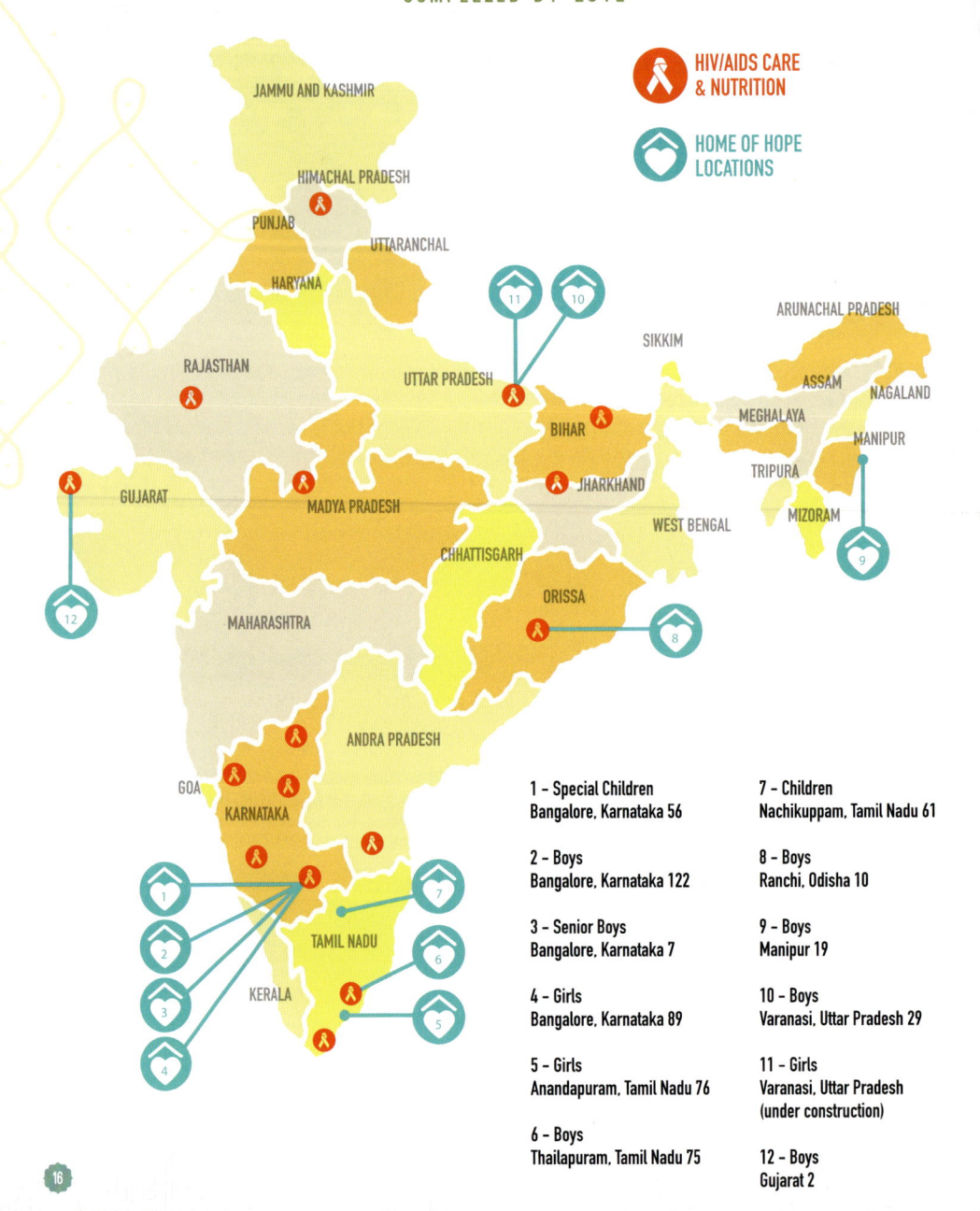

COMPELLED BY LOVE

School time

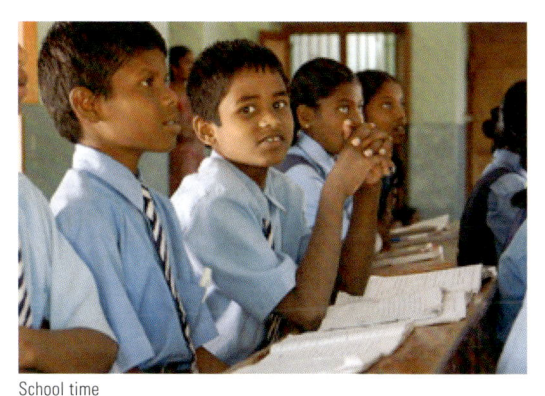

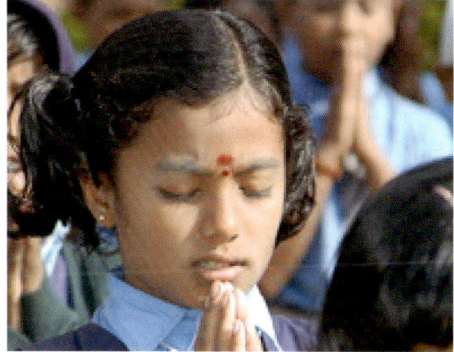

Prayer time

Children's belongings and sleeping area

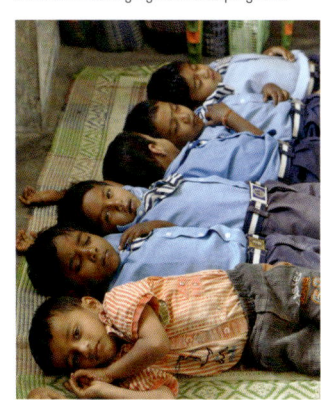

Rest time

A TYPICAL DAY FOR AN INDIAN ORPHAN IN A HOME OF HOPE:

4:45-5:00 am	Wake up
5:00-5:30 am	Prayer
5:30-5:45 am	Coffee
5:45-7:00 am	Personal time
7:00-7:30 am	Morning study
7:30-8:00 am	Breakfast
8:00-8:15 am	Leave for school
8:15 am-4:20 pm	School time
4:20-4:30 pm	Freshen-up
4:30-4:45 pm	Tiffin (snack time)
4:45-5:30 pm	Games
5:30-6:00 pm	Prayer time
6:00-6:30 pm	Personal time
6:30-7:30 pm	Study
7:30-8:00 pm	Dinner
8:00-9:00 pm	Study
9:00 pm	Bed/Lights out

COMPELLED BY LOVE

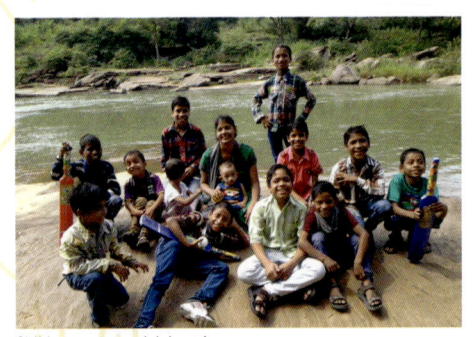

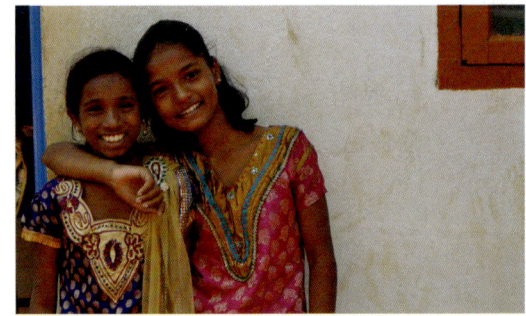

Children on a special day trip

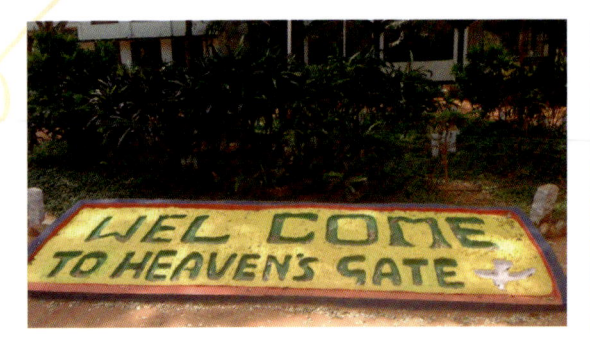

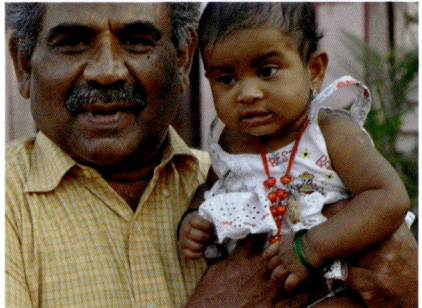

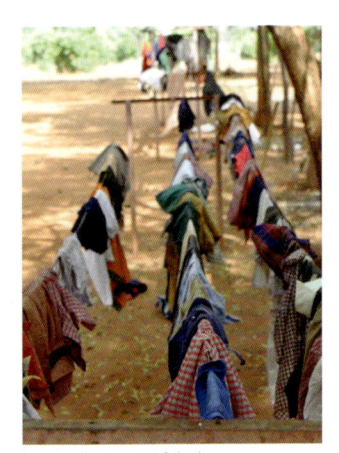

Laundry day at one of the homes

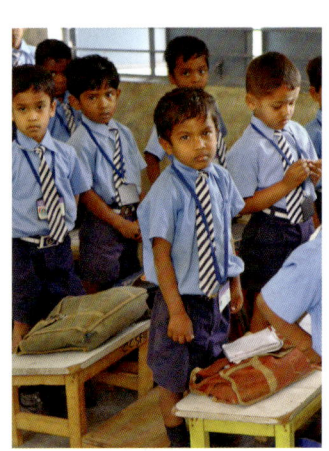

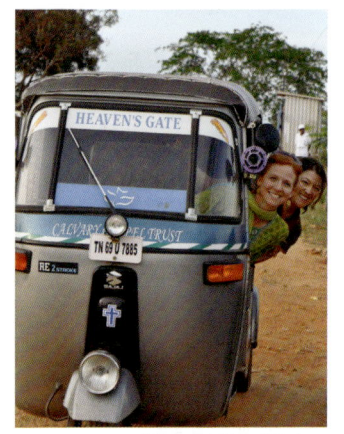

A Heaven's Gate Rickshaw,
a common mode of transportation

COMPELLED BY LOVE

THE NEED BY THE NUMBERS

THE GOVERNMENT OF INDIA ESTIMATES THAT ABOUT 2.4 MILLION INDIANS ARE LIVING WITH HIV

- Children under 15 account for 3.5% of all infections.
- 83% of HIV infections are between 15-49 years.
- Of all HIV infections, 39% are among women (World Bank).
- 36% of people with HIV/AIDS are receiving ART (treatment).

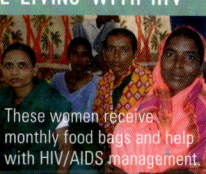

These women receive monthly food bags and help with HIV/AIDS management.

HIV AND AIDS ESTIMATES IN INDIA

DEATHS DUE TO AIDS
130,000 [93,000-160,000] (United Nations)

INDIA

- Home to approximately 1/3 of the world's poor.
- 42% of India, 456 million people, fall below the international poverty line of $1.25 a day.
- Almost 30% of workers are day laborers.
- Only 10% of the population has regular employment.
- 64% of those living in India with the virus do not have access to treatment (Wall Street Journal).
- 42.5% of children in India face malnutrition (New York Times).
- 49% of the world's underweight children live in India (World Health Organization).
- 34% of the world's under developed children live in India (World Health Organization).
- 220,000 children are infected with HIV/AIDS.
- 55,000-60,000 children are born to mothers with HIV/AIDS (without treatment, 30% will become infected).

OUR SPECIAL CHILD IN HOME OF HOPE

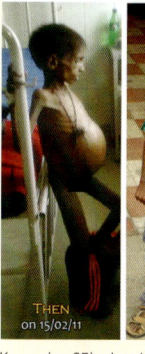

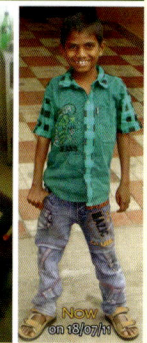

Then on 15/02/11
Now on 18/07/11

Kumar (pg 35) when he arrived at the Home of Hope and the transformation just five months later.

COMPELLED BY LOVE

RUNNING STATS

HALF MARATHON: 13.1 Miles

HEAVEN'S GATE RACES:

Run for the Hills (Fruitland, Idaho)

City of Trees (Boise, Idaho)

Rush Creek Stampede (Cambridge, Idaho)

Heaven's Gate (Boise, Idaho)

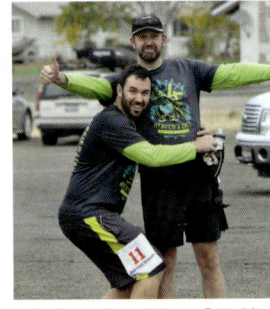

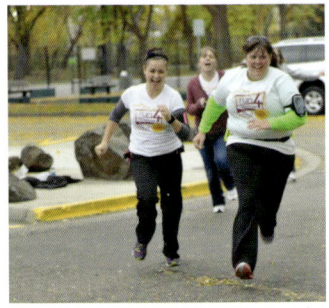

HOW LONG IT TAKES:

John Abernathy and Aaron Catt, 2014

Melissa Bent and Mallory Watson, 2013

Estimated Finish Time for Walkers:

Fast Walkers: 13 minutes/mile (2:50 estimated half marathon time)

Medium Walkers: 15-16 minutes/mile (3:16 estimated half marathon time)

Slower Walkers: 17-19 minutes/mile (3:30 to 3:50 estimated half marathon time)

Estimated Finish Time for Runners:

Fast Paced Runners: 7-9 minutes/mile (1:31 to 2:00 estimated half marathon time)

Medium Paced Runners: 10-11 minutes/mile (2:11 to 2:24 estimated half marathon time)

Slower Paced Runners: 12-14 minutes/mile (2:37 to 3:03 estimated half marathon time)

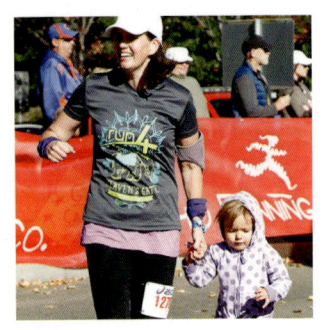

3 year old Delana Hoppock with mom Amy at the finish line

TRAINING:

Most runners and walkers start training 12 weeks prior to the first race. Training includes 3-4 runs during the week and long runs on the weekends that get progressively longer (for example, week 1 long run is 4 miles, week 2 is 5 miles, week 6 is 6 miles, etc.).

FACTS:

- Running burns an average of 975 calories an hour.
- Boosts your immune system
- An estimated 26.5 million Americans run.
- Makes you happier :)
- Half marathon training schedules are easily accessed online.

COMPELLED BY LOVE

FUNDING STATS

"The money is helping the kids. As Run 4 Heaven's Gate has grown and produced more income, the ministry has grown in sync. We've seen a harmonized match of God's timing between the runs and the ministry growth."

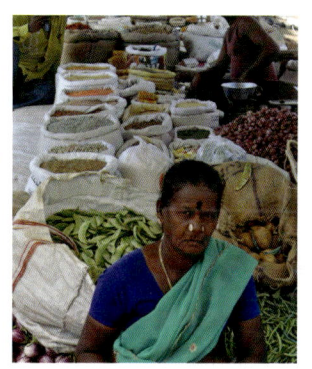

– Pastor Bob Caldwell

An Indian food market

CHARTING THE GROWTH:

Year	Participants	Money Raised
2008	8	Over $13,000
2009	27	$21,442
2010	57	$42,426
2011	76	$64,462
2012	126	$105,219
2013	125	$93,387
2014	148	$159,190
Total So Far	567	$499,126

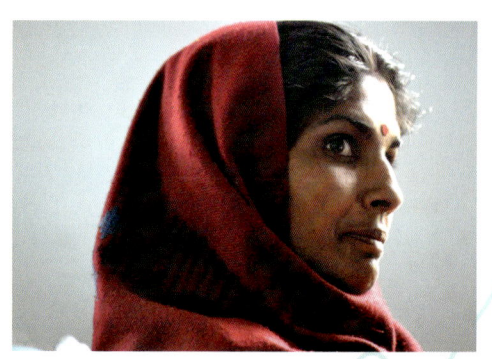

An HIV mom waiting for her monthly nutrition bag

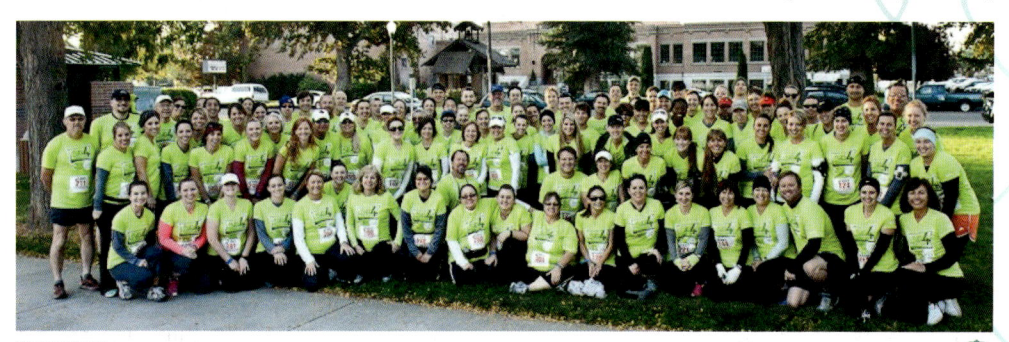

2012 R4HG Team

COMPELLED BY LOVE

RUNNERS REFLECTION: WORDS OF WISDOM AND INSIGHT FROM HEAVEN'S GATE RUNNERS

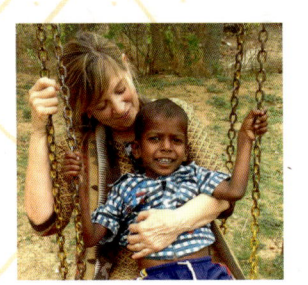

"I've been so humbled and inspired by the love that I've seen from our brother and sisters in India as they reach out to these children and families who have been rejected by others in so many ways, what we do makes a difference. . . it is something little we can do to share in what is already being done, it's a small way we can come along side our brothers and sisters in India."

– CATHY CALDWELL

Cathy Caldwell

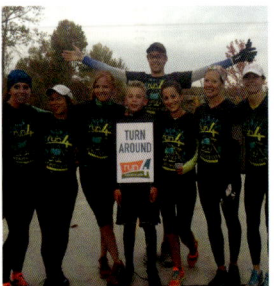

"When I'm running and thinking about the kids in India and what they are going through, I see the truth about my first world problems which are small in the big scheme of things. They seem small in comparison. I think we lose sight of what it is like to fight for survival day in and day out. Running strips away pretense, it's just myself and God: it's so different from my normal day to day life. God provides for our needs when we are out there saying yes."

– BEN MONAGHAN

Ben Monaghan and other runners

"When we were in India with the kids, one of our buses broke down and all the kids and the mission team had to crowd onto one bus. The children made sure that each team member had their own seat. They wouldn't let any team member stand. Our hearts as runners is to serve and sacrifice for the kids, but their heart is the same: to serve us! It's a joy to be a part of it and to see the impact of what we are doing. There is an impact on the community here. I'm honored to be a part of something that is so selfless. It's not about a church, or a person. It's a collective thing. It's what the church should be."

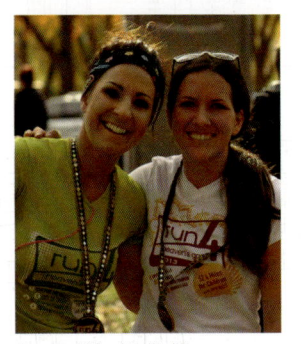

– ANNA MORENO

Anna and friend Hallie Vinson

COMPELLED BY LOVE

"I love running, and it's a joyful privilege to be able to translate my passion for running into an act of worship to my Father in Heaven, as I log mile after mile for His kids in India. What's truly special to me about Run 4 Heaven's Gate, is knowing that all of us who are a part of the team are not only running and walking, but that we're praying for the kids in India the entire time that we're together participating in these four half marathons. It is very special to know that God is hearing all of those prayers being lifted to Him while we're out on that race course together."

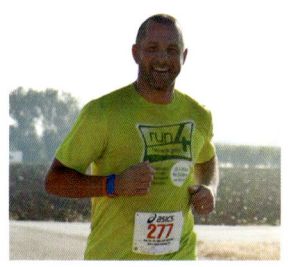

— RYAN STEARNS

Ryan Stearns, 2012

"You have a bond with your Heaven's Gate teammates and feel connected to these people, most likely for the rest of your life. If you want to experience a closer relationship with God, do Heaven's Gate."

— BARRY AND KATHY REISSIG

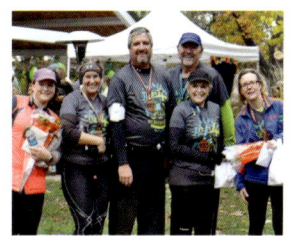

Barry and Kathy Reissig and other runners

"I can do more than I ever thought I could. I have allowed God to use me in whatever ways He wants to, so I just keep stepping out and following. If God wants me to run, then here I am."

— JESSICA HOWIE

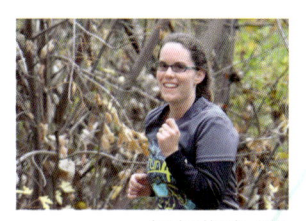

Jessica Howie, 2014

"God calls and brings us through in His way. You don't have to be an athlete. You just have to have a heart and surrender it. For me, it is not an option not to run."

— MELISSA DEL RIO

Melissa Del Rio, 2013

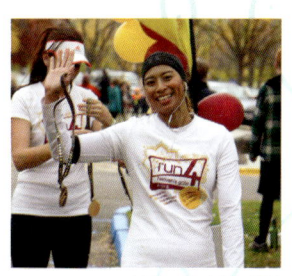

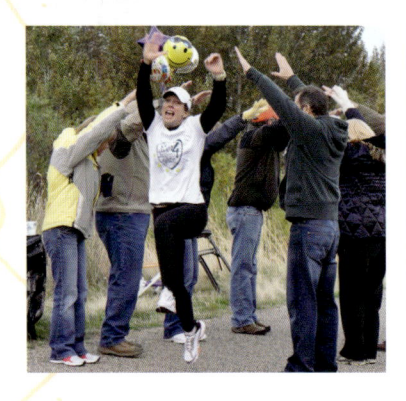

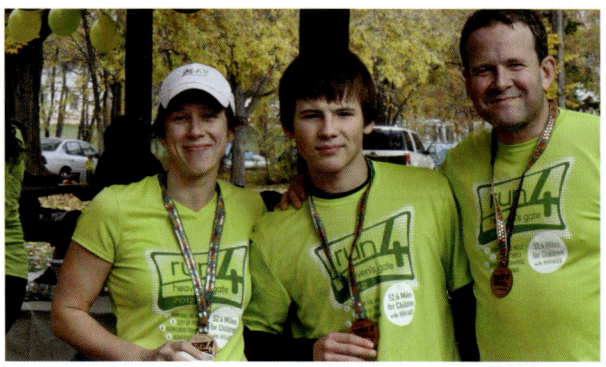

Melinda, Jacob, and Monte Eldfrick, 2013

MELINDA ELDFRICK

Melinda has been on the Run 4 Heaven's Gate team since the beginning. Her bright smile, encouraging words, and contagious zest for life have blessed many runners over the years. "It grows and changes every year. It is fun to see what God has done and to be a part of something so important from the ground up." Melinda is a vital part of the leadership team that supports Dottie. "Melinda helps keep me grounded and she is one of the people I call to pray, and she helps me brainstorm and sort through things that come up." Both women agree that their friendship has been another unexpected benefit and blessing from their commitment to running for children in India.

"It is always a journey. Each year there are different lessons to be learned. I look forward to each year with anticipation." Melinda loves to run and trains regularly. She can complete a half-marathon in under two hours. One year, due to an injury, Melinda had to walk. "It gave me compassion for the commitment of walkers."

What started as a love for running has translated into a family passion and commitment to India. Melinda, her husband, Monte, and teenage son, Jacob, have all taken trips to India to work with the women and children there. "When I went to India, I was overwhelmed by the poverty and disease. But when I saw the people and met the children, they were beautiful. The people are the joy."

Melinda loves her pre-dawn runs with friends. "We talk, we pray, we encourage each other." Some might see running as a physical endeavor, but to Melinda it's a spritual practice as well.

COMPELLED BY LOVE

ANJAMMA

At a train station in the Koppal region of northern Karnataka, a divine appointment took place that changed the trajectory of the Homes of Hope and work of Calvary Chapel Trust in India.

A young mother and her nine-year-old daughter, Anjamma, had just tested positive for HIV at a Calvary Chapel Trust mobile medical outreach near their village. Devastated, they set out to find two strangers who might be able to help: Pastors Bob and Guna. The men were headed to the train station for the twelve-hour journey back to Bangalore. Radhabai, an AIDS widow, knew that Anjamma would face abandonment from their small village when she passed away. Her love compelled Radhabai to find Pastors Bob and Guna, hoping they would be able to help her seemingly hopeless situation.

Bob and Guna were hearing more and more about the spread of HIV/AIDS among the poor. When they were faced with what to do for this desperate mother, they knew that helping even one family might open a door for many others. Setting their doubts aside, they asked them to come to Bangalore for more testing. Anjamma's mother made a courageous decision to take a journey farther than she had ever gone before. It demonstrated the lengths she was willing to go for her precious daughter. Once in Bangalore, further testing confirmed their positive diagnoses for HIV/AIDS.

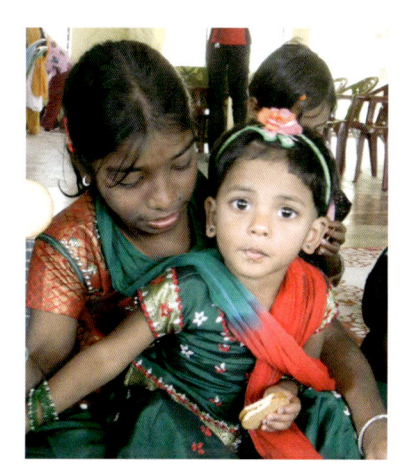

Of that decision Pastor Bob recalls, "God gave us the gift of faith to believe that He would show us a way. We feared that our homes might be shut down because of prejudice, but instead, doors we never could have imagined opened. God has provided all we've needed for every single child that has come to us."

Today, Anjamma is a student hoping to become a doctor, she loves to dance, and the caregivers report that her belief in Jesus keeps her going.

COMPELLED BY LOVE

MIKE SLAUGHTER

FAVORITE BIBLE VERSE: Jeremiah 29:11 (NLT) "For I know the plans I have for you, says the Lord. They are plans for good and not for evil, to give you a future and a hope."

FAVORITE PLACE TO RUN: Stanley, ID

HIDDEN TALENT: Spinning Tops

BEST ADVICE: Run smarter, not harder.

LISTENS TO WHILE RUNNING: Toby Mac

A lifelong runner, Mike has had a longstanding goal of competing in the Boston Marathon. So, when he heard about the idea of Run 4 Heaven's Gate the first year, it was easy for him to commit to being on the team. Mike has been a part of the R4HG team each year, but it hasn't always been a given that he would be able to run.

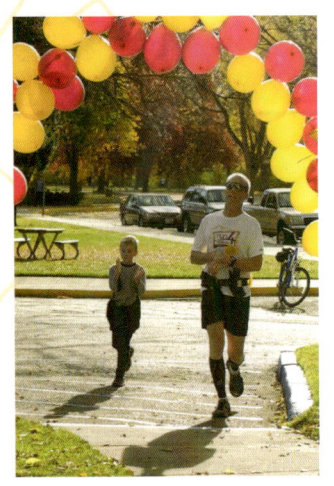

Mike Slaughter with son, 2014

After several attempts to qualify for the Boston Marathon, he sustained an injury that he thought might cause him to hang up his running shoes for good. "I knew I couldn't run Boston with my injury and after the last Heaven's Gate race that year, I told my wife I was retiring from running. My leg wasn't getting better. It was getting worse. I didn't see any future for me as a runner."

Mike's retirement from running only lasted about six months. "I got the email about signing up for Run 4 Heaven's Gate that year and I started thinking, 'Maybe I can do this.'" He woke up early the next morning, found his running shoes, and ran one mile. "My leg didn't hurt. I thought, 'I'll do the races again this year, even if I have to walk them.' It felt like a miracle. The fact that God cared enough about me to let me be able to do what I enjoy *and* to be a part of helping orphans in India is a testimony to His grace."

Mike ran all the races that year and continued momentum with his training. He ran the Boston Marathon in 2013, the year of the marathon bombing. He had crossed the finish line by the time the bomb went off.

Mike says, "You've got to get to the end of your ability and put your trust in God. There is no way I could do this by myself."

COMPELLED BY LOVE

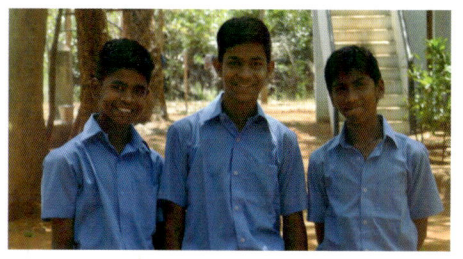

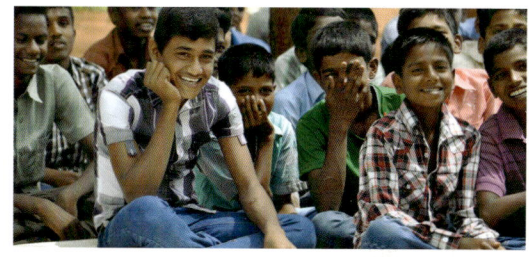

Anand, Thayappa, and Manjunath

THREE FRIENDS

Anand, Thayappa, and Manjunath are three friends who have walked the path of abandonment, fear, mistreatment, and loneliness through their separate lives. They also have found hope, acceptance, love, and purpose in the Home of Hope.

These three young men met when they came to the home in their early teen years. Each boy lost at least one parent to AIDS. One's father murdered his mother when he was just four years old, another became an orphan when both parents died, and another was discarded when a new stepfather came into his mother's life. They should have been under the protective care and nurture of parents who loved them, but were instead thrust into a difficult and dangerous world to fend for themselves, alone.

Each boy struggled to survive in unfriendly and dangerous situations. The challenges they faced have left scars that each is still dealing with in their own way.

In a hopeless world, hope found each boy.

Anand was found alone in a busy train station in Bangalore.

Manjunath was rescued from child labor abuse.

Thayappa came from another orphanage.

The Home of Hope is truly an oasis of peace and healing in these young men's lives.

These, like many other HIV positive children in the Home of Hope, have to come to terms with their past and deal with fear about their future. Each time one of their friends lose their life to AIDS it reminds everyone of the fragility and uncertainty of their own. Each boy is receiving vocational training in agriculture. Additionally, Thayappa is known as a man of prayer and is studying the Bible diligently with hopes of serving in the Home of Hope.

COMPELLED BY LOVE

KATIE PEW

FAVORITE BIBLE VERSE: 1 Samuel 12:24 (NASB) "Only fear the Lord, and serve Him in truth with all your heart; for consider what great things He has done for you."

FAVORITE PLACE TO RUN: Boise Foothills and anytime I go on vacation, as it's a great way to see a new place.

BEST ADVICE: Remember why you love to run and don't get distracted with the rest.

HIDDEN TALENT: Having the courage to try new things.

HYDRATES WITH: When I don't have coffee in hand, I generally stick to water.

Katie Pew and Melissa Del Rio at the Heaven's Gate Half Marathon finish 2013

After her third baby, Katie was looking for a way to get back in shape. She heard about Run 4 Heaven's Gate and thought running four half marathons would be a good way to achieve her goal. What started out as an opportunity to stay fit quickly turned into a personal passion and a cause that unites her family. "My heart changed 180 degrees during the first season I ran. Running became a way to work out my faith and be connected to the Lord." As Katie and her family have seen the impact they are able to make with friends, family, and most importantly the children in India, participating in the Heaven's Gate races every year is not a question or consideration. It's simply what her family does.

Supporting the kids in India has become a family focus. "My kids ride their bikes while I train, they cheer me on at the races, they show me grace if I have to miss a game for a race." Her children love to share about the orphans in India with their homeschool co-op and have organized Otter Pop sales and jog-a-thons to raise awareness and money. "We are all gifted with something. Running is a gift. I love being able to share with my kids that when God gives you a talent—a gift—you can use what you love to glorify the Lord. I want to show my kids that as we are faithful to use our talents, God uses these gifts to further His kingdom."

"I can run. I can't give thousands of dollars myself, but I can run 52.4 miles and hopefully inspire others to use their passions for God's bigger purpose."

COMPELLED BY LOVE

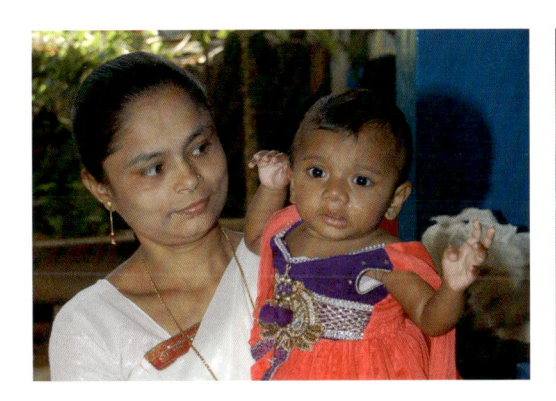

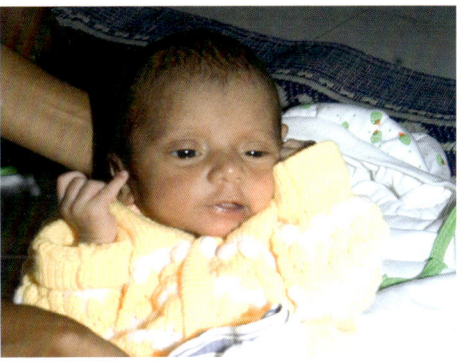

NIRMALA

Nirmala was found crying on the steps of a prayer chapel in Bangalore when she was just ten days old. Shortly thereafter, officials gave Nirmala to Calvary Chapel Trust to care for. Many questions remain unanswered about Nirmala's past. Was there a loving family nearby searching for their little one? If not, why was she abandoned? Once she was put under Calvary Chapel Trust's care she was given an initial health exam where it was determined that the child was HIV positive. This provided some answers to why she had been abandoned. Poor families are simply unable to care for a sick child. Coupled with fear and social stigma, this ensured that no one was coming to reclaim their daughter. The emotional pain of abandonment is added to the long list of things an infected child must bear.

Infants admitted into the Home of Hope are placed in the home for girls in Bangalore. When Nirmala arrived, she was given an exclusive caregiver named Priya. Priya cares for all of Nirmala's needs just as a mother would. She feeds, baths, plays with, and rocks her to sleep at night. Additionally, Nirmala is raised within the community; it's the Indian way. It is not uncommon to find a baby bouncing on the hip of an older "sister" in the home. Each child is nurtured and loved by all.

Priya, Nirmala's caregiver, has her own sad story of abandonment. She was a married to a migrant worker at the tender age of thirteen and had three sons. Her husband contracted HIV, which eventually claimed his life, but not before he passed it on to his young bride. Because of HIV, she was cast out of her community, but has since found a purpose for her life as a caregiver at the Home of Hope. Priya and Nirmala have found both a home and hope.

COMPELLED BY LOVE

MELISSA DEL RIO

FAVORITE BIBLE VERSE: Isaiah 40:31 (ESV) "But they who wait for the Lord shall renew their strength; they shall mount up with wings like eagles; they shall run and not be weary; they shall walk and not faint."

FAVORITE PLACE TO RUN: Red Cliff Trail at Camels Back Park

HIDDEN TALENT: I can eat more food than a guy twice my size.

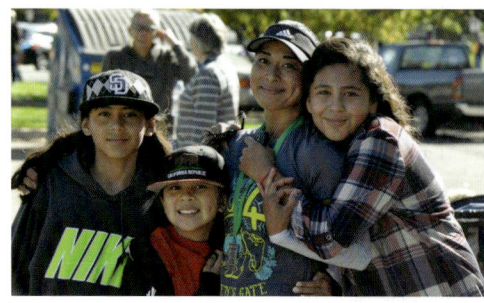

Melissa Del Rio and her children at the finish line

BEST ADVICE: Don't let your circumstances define your life. Trust in God's love and faithfulness. His plans for us are always so much greater than our own.

LISTENS TO WHILE RUNNING: Reggae, R&B, and Rap

When Melissa committed to running for Heaven's Gate she didn't realize the impact that decision would have on her family. After years of hearing about Run 4 Heaven's Gate, Melissa realized she didn't really have a reason not to run. But then, just a few weeks before her first race, she severely injured her IT band. "It felt like someone was taking a hammer to my IT band. I ran eight miles of the first race and started crying. I realized it wasn't about me and how I finished. The purpose (running for the kids in India) was still the same no matter how I finished."

In the year that followed, Melissa's first Run 4 Heaven's Gate season, her life came crashing down. Her husband of 18 years told her he was leaving, she experienced severe breathing problems, and her three children were dealing with feelings of abandonment in light of their father's absence. As a new chapter dawned in Melissa's life, the call to Run 4 Heaven's Gate remained the same.

"My kids went with me to the kick-off meeting for that next season. They all started crying as they watched the video of kids in India. My kids related at a heart level with the feeling of abandonment that the kids in India feel and my kids feel too." From that moment on, running Heaven's Gate became a family affair. "God has woven our hearts together with a united purpose to help the orphans in India. My kids see the children in India as their brothers and sisters. As we have had to redefine family, the kids in India have become a very real part of our family." Melissa's kids go with her on training runs, they cheer her on at the races, share their mom's progress on Facebook, and make sure she recovers well from each race. Melissa has found that in the midst of suffering and pain, God is faithful. He gives her joy and the assurance that His love never fails.

COMPELLED BY LOVE

SANJIT

"The doctors had given up hope for Sanjit," Brother Henry recalled, "but God's plan was different and He kept him alive for a reason."

Sanjit shares his story in his own words:

> "I am from a Muslim family, from a place called Deoria near Varanasi. My dad passed away when I was born and I have never seen him. I came to know that my father was drinking too much alcohol which led to his death. My mother passed away when I was two years old from depression. I have no proper memory of my childhood. Only after I was diagnosed with HIV/AIDS, I came to know that my parents died of this same disease. For twelve years I was brought up by my Aunt Kathaija, along with her children. I was not given proper care in my aunt's house and I was getting very sick often. I had become very lean.
>
> I was admitted to the Home of Hope where I am very happy and experience the love of Jesus. God has been leading me all these years. It has been three years since I came to the Home of Hope, Asha Sadan. I often get severe fevers, vomiting, and diarrhea and am admitted to various hospitals. My CD4 count (a marker for white blood cells) has come down. God strengthens me and gives me life. Even though I came to the home in 6th grade, I was unable to complete school due to my sickness.
>
> I have memorized more than 80 Bible verses and these promises make me strong. I spend time reading the Word of God. I help younger children in their studies, clean the house, help in accounts, and teach songs and stories. I am doing well now and have increased my weight. For the past two months I have not had vomiting or diarrhea. Praise Jesus!"

Henry, the director for the Varanasi Home of Hope, says, "Sanjit is a living testimony to the staff, children, and sponsors of God's love and grace. He is very healthy and active now."

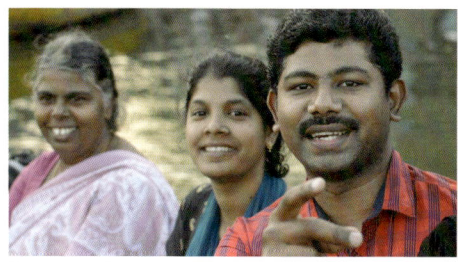

Henry, Pastor Guna's son, and director of the Varanasi Home of Hope, 2013

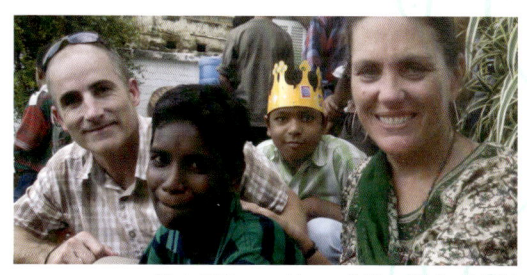

Marty Williams and Lauren Phillips with Sanjit, 2014

COMPELLED BY LOVE

DAVE AND LINDA WILHITE

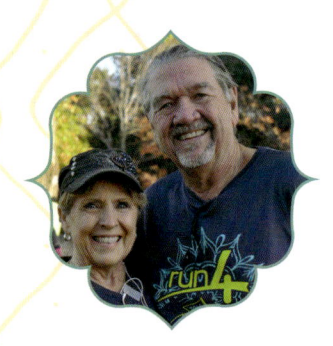

FAVORITE PLACE TO RUN: Boise Greenbelt and foothills trails

BEST ADVICE: Train hard.

HIDDEN TALENT: Soul sloshing… It just means meeting people one on one and talking about the deep things of life. (It's best done at a coffee house!)

"At our age, our goal was to run for Heaven's Gate without running through it."

Dave Wilhite's famous words have inspired and challenged more runners than maybe any other Heaven's Gate runner ever. This couple who in their mid-60s are an inspiration to their fellow runner and walkers, their friends and family who faithfully support them, and the children in India who benefit from their dedication.

When they decided to participate several years ago, they were among the oldest team members. "I didn't even know how long a half-marathon was when I signed up," Dave laughed. He had recently lost 100 pounds and walking was part of his motivation to keep the weight off. Quickly, both he and Linda realized that the physical benefits were only a small part of the Run 4 Heaven's Gate experience. The Wilhites trained with a local run/walk training program, and as Dave puts it, "We did everything exactly as they told us to!"

"At first, it was all about my bucket list and staying active," admitted Linda. "As I trained and especially during the half marathons, I would think that even though this was extremely difficult for me, it is a small sacrifice on my part for the children in India. This God-inspired mindset keeps me putting one foot in front of the other."

"From a purely logical standpoint, we realize that we should probably 'act our age' and not run, but as long as we can, it's a sacrifice we are willing to make to help these children," Dave and Linda both agree.

"We've seen over the years that we can do more by running/walking than we could ever do on our own. We can't go to India and we can't give large amounts of money, but we can do this."

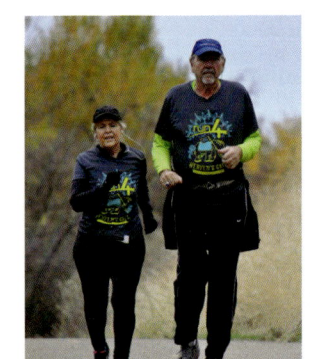

Dave and Linda Wilhite inspiring all the runners with their dedication and joy

COMPELLED BY LOVE

IN MEMORY OF ARUL

Arul was a friendly boy who enjoyed everyone, loved to help the other children, and had many friends at the Home of Hope for Boys, Bangalore. He used his skills whenever he could, even volunteering to move to Varanasi to help start a new Home of Hope for children with HIV. He spoke Hindi fluently and helped the children and staff from southern India learn the language while he interpreted and translated. Arul was a young man of prayer and was known to spend many hours in personal time with God.

At the age of fifteen, Arul came to live in the Home of Hope after he was diagnosed with HIV. His family members could no longer afford the anti-retroviral medicines that he needed to combat the deadly disease.

While in Varanasi, Arul fell sick and was diagnosed with sputum tuberculosis and severe dysentery which caused his health to deteriorate quickly. Pastor Guna and Victoria spent two hours praying with him until he died. His last word was "Yesappa" (meaning Jesus, Father).

Although his life was cut short by the effects of AIDS, Arul left a lasting legacy—one of unshakeable commitment to prayer and the joy he found when using his gifts and talents to serve others. We remember Arul as a young man who, though very sick himself, was instrumental in starting the Home of Hope in Varanasi.

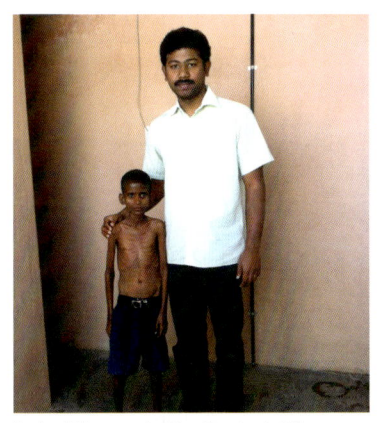

Arul and Henry worked together to start the Varanasi Home of Hope.

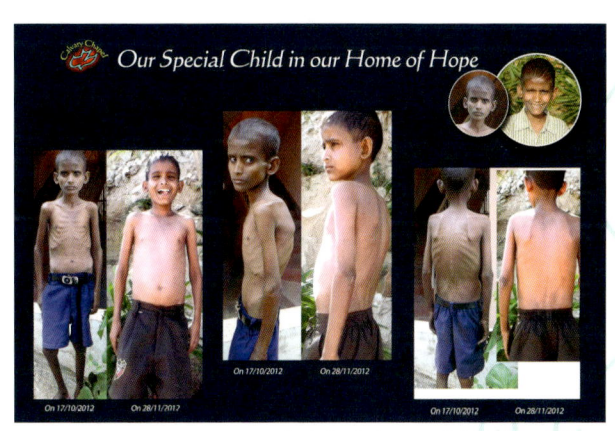

Arul after just one month in the Home of Hope.

COMPELLED BY LOVE

TERIANN LUKEHART

BEST ADVICE: Treat all people the way you want all people to treat you.

HIDDEN TALENT: Drawing and painting

LISTENS TO WHILE RUNNING: I listen to nothing, then I can pray and I listen to the sound of my footsteps. It's very tranquil.

HYDRATES WITH: Water is the best! Unless I am training for half marathons, then I need something with electrolytes.

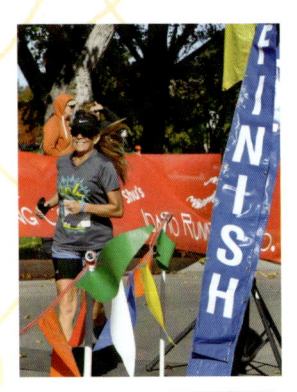

TeriAnn Lukehart crossing the City of Trees Half Marathon finish line 2014

As a lifelong athlete who competed in track at the collegiate level, winning was commonplace. "I had trophies and awards in everything," TeriAnn recalled. "I heard about Run 4 Heaven's Gate from Dottie the very first year they ran. I was tired of training and competition after a lifetime of training for myself. I didn't think that I could do it." Additionally, as a sprinter and hurdler, distances were out of her comfort zone. For several years she heard about the races but never seriously considered participating… Until, like many others, TeriAnn's family was hit hard by the recession. "We lost everything."

At that low point in her life, she felt God calling her to Run 4 Heaven's Gate. With a body and mind that were broken and tired from years of competition and the financial stress her family was under, she made the decision to trust God and run not for herself, but for Him. "I trusted God for the training, words to say in the fundraising letter, my race entry fees, and for running shoes. I was running for Him, not for myself. It changed my heart."

"I was a different person when I crossed the finish line of the first half marathon. It was the first time in my sports history that I had relied on Jesus and not myself. It was so emotional."

Now, she runs every year and can't imagine not doing so. "God has opened my eyes to see the needs in the world. He has shown me that if I'm willing and will allow God, He will equip me. Running for Heaven's Gate is one great way to help people and really make a difference."

COMPELLED BY LOVE

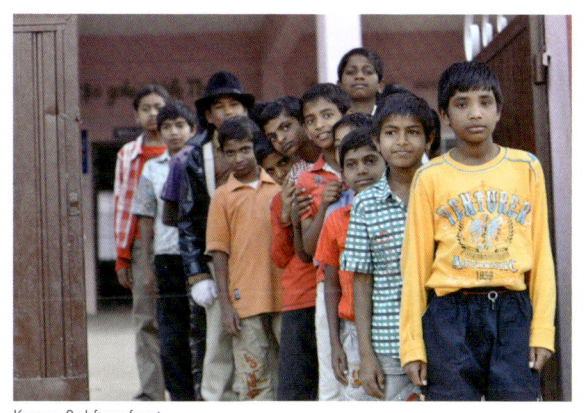

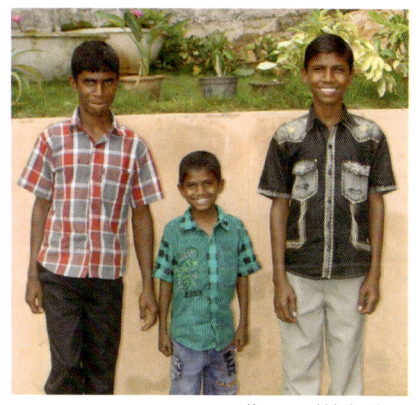

Kumar, 3rd from front

Kumar and his brothers

IN MEMORY OF KUMAR

Kumar came to live in the Home of Hope when he was eleven years old. His father had passed away from AIDS, so his mother made the difficult decision to leave Kumar and his two brothers in the care of others. She later became very sick and passed away.

Kumar was born with HIV, which made it difficult for him to pursue any academics. He was often sick and many times doctors believed he would not survive but he always proved them wrong and recovered. At the homes in Bangalore and Varanasi, he was friendly and well-liked by the other children and caregivers and was often willing to make sacrifices of himself so other children could benefit. He loved cycling, boating, drawing, and playing cricket, and was often seen praying by himself.

Kumar fought many hard battles during his short life until abdominal tuberculosis finally claimed him. Pastor Guna and Victoria were at his bedside for many days preceding his death. When it became apparent that Kumar would not recover this time, Guna asked him what he would like to have. Instead of a toy, candy, or a favorite meal, Kumar asked for one very precious thing, that Victoria would hold him in her arms. When she did, he was able to finally rest in peace in the arms of the woman he came to know as *amma*.

Kumar's life was too short, but his wide smile, friendly attitude, and vigor with which he fought against the trials he faced, proving doctors wrong time and again, still encourage all who knew him.

RIGHT: Cathy, Kumar, and Dottie, 2011

COMPELLED BY LOVE

VANESSA MCCRORY

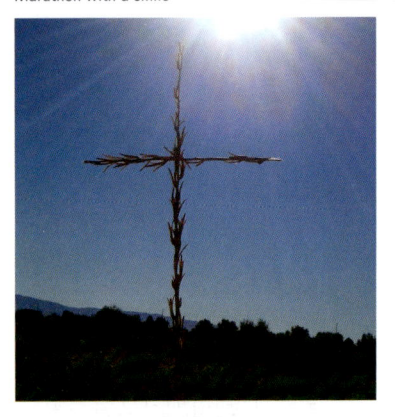

"I don't have time for this; my life is falling apart." Vanessa thought when she heard about the upcoming Run 4 Heaven's Gate season.

During the summer of 2014, Vanessa's family was seriously struggling. In the middle of her grief over a family member's experience with mental illness and drug abuse, she knew that God wanted her to Run 4 Heaven's Gate. As she started to train, she saw crosses everywhere: plants along the route, sticks on the path, and vapor trails in the sky, all reminding her that Jesus was with her and she wasn't alone. God knew that running would be a much needed way to cope with stress and a source of spiritual encouragement through the trials she was facing.

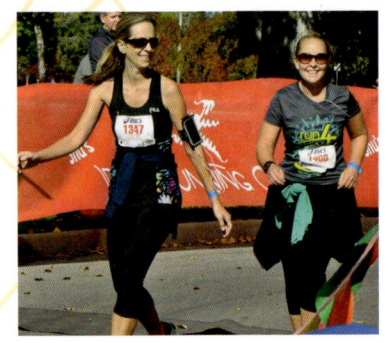

Vanessa McCrory finishing the City of Trees Half Marathon with a smile

#JESUSRUNSWITHYOU

The days leading up to her first Run 4 Heaven's Gate race were some of the saddest and loneliest days for Vanessa and her two young girls. "The first two miles of her first race were the hardest of the 52.4 miles. I was ready physically, just not emotionally for the races to come. So much was going on in our lives and it was beginning to take a toll." Before mile two, Vanessa had to stop and pray, "Lord help me. Help me do this for you. Please work all the horrible things in my life for your glory."

"I heard His ever calming voice say to me; 'Okay, Ness. Just one foot in front of the other. You got this.'"

At the end of the race, Vanessa discovered the one and only text she has ever received from her mom, which read: "#jesusrunswithyou."

"I opened it and cried like a baby. Jesus ran all 52.4 miles with me and He didn't stop after that. He keeps me going, motivated, and runs daily with me. He has never left me. He is Good."

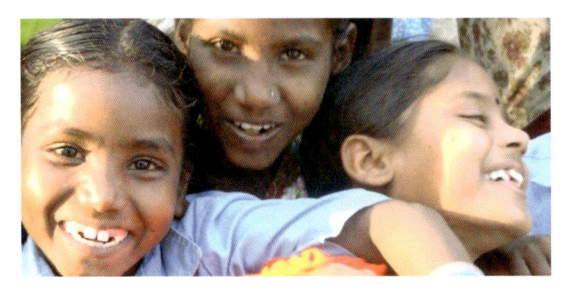

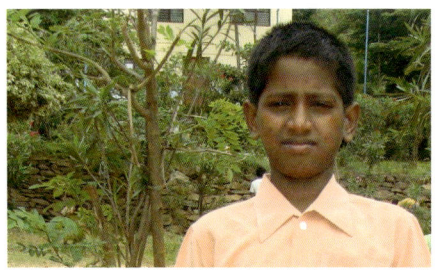

RAMA

Rama's life had been marked by running—but always by running away—until he ran into the Home of Hope in Bangalore.

Rama never knew his father, and his mother died when he was in sixth grade. An orphan alone in the world, he was put in a hostel where he daily endured verbal and physical abuse. Rama ran away. He got a job feeding cows, but the cows were fed better than he was (and treated better too), so Rama ran. He got a job working at a kennel feeding dogs but an accident landed Rama in the hospital where it was discovered that he had HIV. With this virus and no family, Rama was sent to live in a home for children who had committed crimes.

"This place was like a jail and I was not allowed to go outside the campus. As they found out that I had HIV, I was discriminated against and was feeling very lonely. I was treated like an untouchable and had separate plate and glass. After spending four months in this place, I was referred to Home of Hope, Calvary Chapel, Bangalore."

At the Home of Hope, Rama's life changed. "Right from the first day I experienced the love of God in this place. The staff and children were very friendly and there was not a sign of discrimination. I never felt so loved in my life. I came to know about Jesus Christ and started reading the Bible. I was put in the 9th grade, but I was unable to perform well in school as it had been a long time since I last attended so I opted to do gardening work and became an assistant to the driver in the home."

"My desire is to make other children like me to be happy."

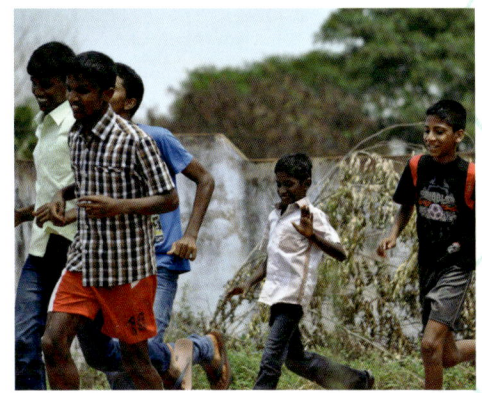

COMPELLED BY LOVE

TERRYL LIIMAKKA

A slow and painful walk in her neighborhood was the beginning of Terryl's Run 4 Heaven's Gate journey. "I had injured my back and was in a back brace. The physical pain was so great that I didn't even want to get out of bed, which isn't like me at all!" That difficult walk in the unusual February sunshine was not only a physical, but emotional, and spiritual turning point in Terryl's life.

When just a month later she saw the video announcement about the upcoming Run 4 Heaven's Gate season, she knew she needed to be a part of the team. "I love children and I've always loved India. As I watched the video, I felt the Lord say to me 'If you can walk, you can do this, I want you to do this.'"

"I followed a local run/walk training group schedule and slowly increased my mileage in the months leading up to my first Heaven's Gate race. I loved the training. It was beautiful and it wasn't a major sacrifice. I'm not a runner, I'm a walker, and I always felt better after the training walks!" Terryl says with a smile.

Terryl's husband supported her by going on training walks with her three nights a week. Her second grade class also got involved in supporting their beloved teacher and sharing hope with kids in India. "The kids put a jar on my desk, and many of my students emptied their piggy banks to help support the kids in India. We prayed daily as a class for the children in the Home of Hope."

One season wasn't enough for Terryl and during her second season, her teenage daughter joined the team. "I had more pain and injuries that season. I couldn't go as fast. The slower pace allowed me to meet more people and build new relationships with other Heaven's Gate team members. It was all about the relationships with other walkers that year!"

What started out as a dark season of physical pain ended in contagious hope impacting Terryl, her family, her classroom, and lives of children in India.

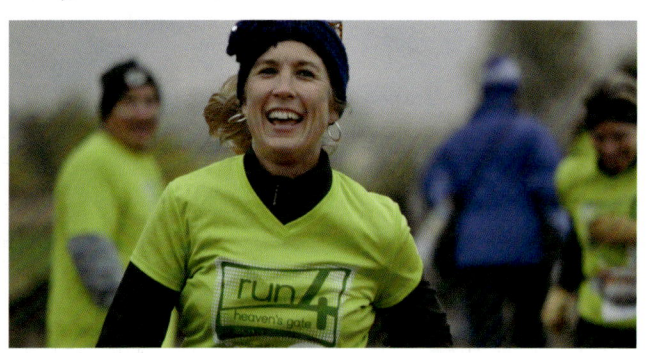

Terryl Liimakka finishing with joy, 2013

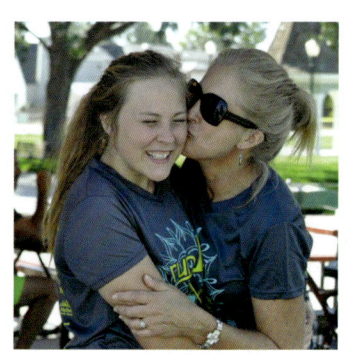

Terryl and daughter Shaelyn, 2014

COMPELLED BY LOVE

IN MEMORY OF SHIVA

Shiva lost his life to AIDS, but not before he experienced love living in the Home of Hope where he learned to share this love with other children. Shiva enjoyed helping younger children with their chores, homework, and reading. He was a good student, knew many Bible verses, and had a passion for prayer.

He came to the home when he was just ten years old. After losing both of his parents to AIDS, he was sent to live with his extended family who mistreated and isolated him. Once in the Home of Hope in Varanasi, he was able to attend school, make friends, and grow physically, spiritually, and emotionally.

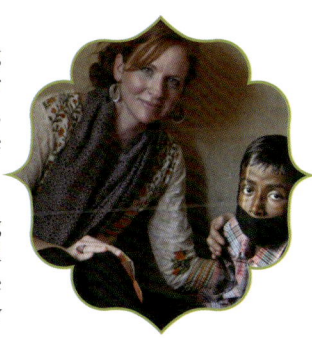

Dottie and Shiva, 2013

Shiva's health declined quickly when he was diagnosed with Tuberculosis and Slim's Disease, which caused prolonged fever and weight loss. In February 2014, he passed away peacefully with his Home of Hope family by his side.

Dottie, who met Shiva in March 2013, wrote, "Little Shiva was dying. He looked very sick, was wearing a black mask, and sitting on his little cot on a concrete floor. He was literally skin and bones, and had sores inside his mouth. It was truly one of the most difficult moments I've ever experienced. As we prayed with him, I held his little hand in mine. To be with a child so close to death was heartbreaking. I couldn't help thinking of my own girls. The thought of them having to endure even a day of what had been Shiva's life was unbearable, yet, I was so thankful that Shiva was able to spend his last few months in our orphanage. He was loved, nourished, and went to school. He got to be a child—an experience he only knew for a short time during his young life. He was able to die with dignity, knowing he was loved, knowing that he had value."

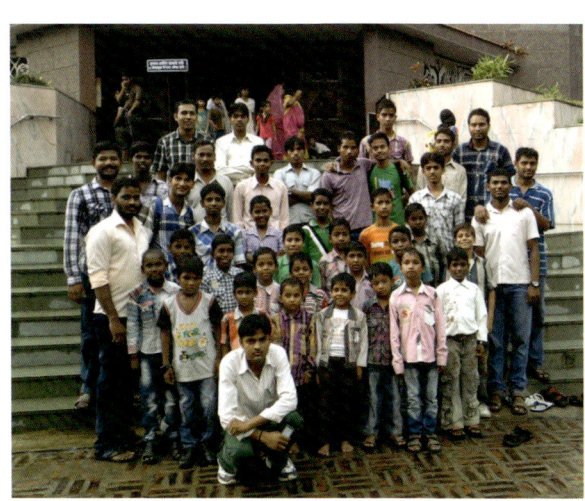

Home of Hope, Varanasi

COMPELLED BY LOVE

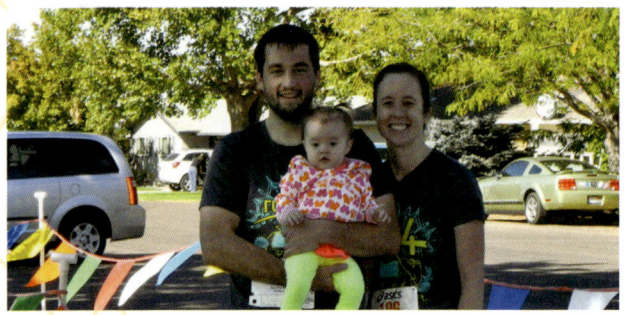

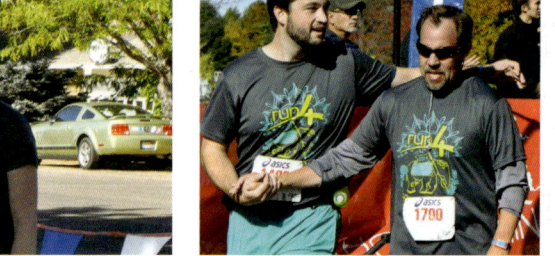

Josiah, Kim, and Eliana Peters. R4HG is a family affair.

Josiah Peters finishing with Mike Westover

JOSIAH AND KIM PETERS

While out for a bike ride, Josiah was hit by a truck two weeks before his second Run 4 Heaven's Gate season. "I had been looking forward to the second year of Run 4 Heaven's Gate. I just completed a half iron man race and was in the best shape of my life going into that season. I was looking forward to setting a personal record (PR), but overnight it went from the year to set a PR to asking myself if I could even finish. I learned so much that year." Josiah reflected. "It set my priorities straight. It wasn't about me or my physical abilities; it was about the kids. I met so many people walking that I wouldn't have met if I was running for a PR."

Josiah has run every year since his first season, accompanied by his wife Kim several of those years. In many ways, their life is shaped by the Heaven's Gate season. "We send support letters to Kim's family in Louisiana and it's a way that we can share our hearts and the things that really matter to us."

The most recent race was a family affair. Their 10 month old daughter Eliana, sporting her own Run 4 Heaven's Gate race shirt and running shoes, rode in a stroller for every race. "She only missed the last two miles of the first race because we got a flat tire and grandparents were able to rescue her so we could finish." The Peters are a young family orienting their life around spreading hope and doing meaningful things together.

"We couldn't make a bigger impact in 12-15 hours (the amount of time they spend running the 4 half marathons) than we can running Heaven's Gate."

COMPELLED BY LOVE

BEN AND CHRISTINE MONAGHAN

As a competitive road cyclist, Ben was used to rigorous training schedules and the discipline required to achieve challenging physical goals. Ben's mom, Christine, was always happy to support her son, but training and running half marathons was not her passion. Ben knew that he wanted to be on the team and he was eager to share the experience with his mom. "Ben was dropping hints every other day," Christine recalled. "I had no desire to do this. I was happy to support him and others, but it wasn't what I wanted to do."

It was on a walk that Christine reflected on some advice she often shared with her five kids, "Don't miss your potential because you are afraid to try something." Christine realized that she needed to follow her own advice. "Once I saw the bigger picture—supporting the kids in India—it became more about the cause and less about the physical challenge. I knew I could do it for those kids."

With Ben as her trainer and coach, the mom and son team started training. Their already close relationship blossomed and changed to an even closer one. "I had to trust my son as my trainer and take his advice about resting and pushing myself. He knew what he was doing. He is a good coach."

It was a physical challenge for Christine to run the races. "I learned there are so many parallels to life that can be learned through running. There are times in the race when you feel good and times when you are so worn down you don't think you can go on. When I ran eleven miles for the first time, I didn't think I could go any further, but then Everlasting God by Lincoln Brewster came on about renewing strength through waiting on the Lord. I was baffled to have my spirit so light in something so physically draining. At that moment, I experienced the spiritual overriding the physical." Running brought new clarity and insight in unexpected ways for Christine.

Ben and Christine ran the last race in the Heaven's Gate series together. "We got to reflect on the six months of training together with the same goal. It was an emotional and sweet time for us."

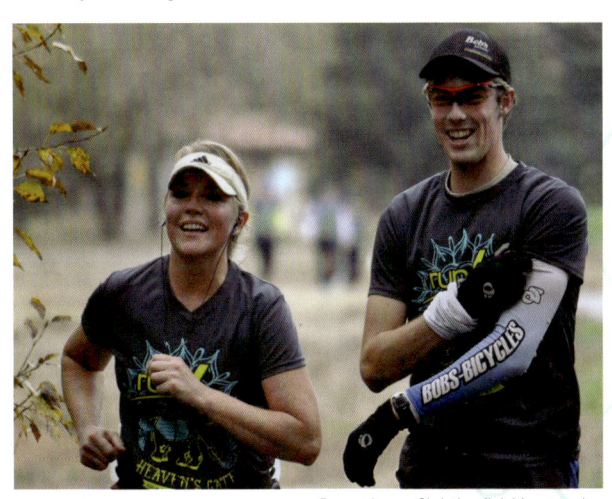

Ben and mom Christine finishing together

COMPELLED BY LOVE

CAMILLE LEVI

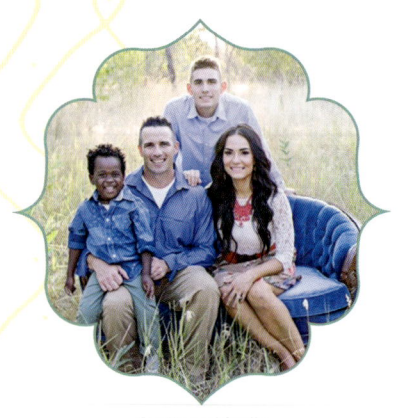

Camille and family

FAVORITE BIBLE VERSE: James 1:27 (NKJV) "Pure and undefiled religion before God and the Father is this: to visit orphans and widows in their trouble, and to keep oneself unspotted from the world."

FAVORITE PLACE TO RUN: Boise Foothills, or anywhere with friends

BEST ADVICE: Start a training program early and increase gradually!

Camille had planned to skip the ten-mile run with her local training group. The day before, Camille found out she was facing her fifth miscarriage. Overwhelmed by heartache and sadness, she wanted to sleep in, but woke up early, and faithfully laced up her running shoes. Putting on her big sunglasses to hide her tears, she planned to go do the training and keep to herself. When she arrived, her fellow Run 4 Heaven's Gate teammates noticed something was wrong and surrounded her with love and fellowship. "I am tied together with those women because of that run. We talked; we prayed. God had perfectly put together that group. Many of those women had experienced the same heartache that I was going through."

"As I did the training and Run 4 Heaven's Gate races that year, I was able to pray though all of the trials in my life. I used all of that time alone running to pray, to sing, to memorize verses. It was during that time that my husband's heart was changed and we began to move forward with adopting our son."

Camille found, as many Run 4 Heaven's Gate team members do, that through the running and sacrifice of love she was making for the kids in India, her own healing began.

"We set limits on ourselves and God, and when we overcome physical limitations, it opens the door to what God can do in and through us. There is a much bigger purpose than you can ever imagine."

Camille has gone on to adopt two sons, run for Mrs. Idaho, and complete her first marathon.

COMPELLED BY LOVE

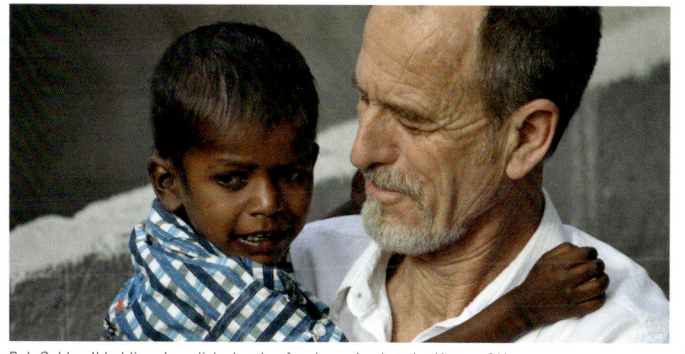

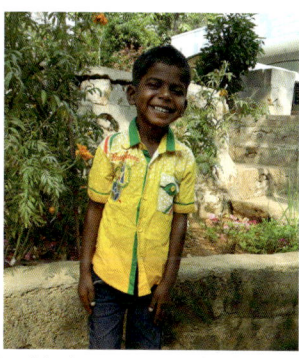

Bob Caldwell holding Jagadish shortly after he arrived at the Home of Hope

Jagadish after one year in the Home of Hope

JAGADISH

Jagadish was abandoned near the Shuttle Goods Terminal, at a busy train station in Bangalore. Amidst the hustle, dirt, and chaos, an ill four-year-old boy was found abandoned and alone. Once officials found that the child's medical tests revealed he was HIV positive, he was placed into the care of the Home of Hope in Bangalore. His physical and mental health was precarious, but after the appropriate treatment, great love, and attentive care, Jagadish's health began to improve. It wasn't easy for Jagadish, but slowly he found peace, accepted love, and made friends.

We don't know much about the past of Jagadish before he came into the care of Home of Hope. It's safe to guess that poverty, sickness, and overwhelming hopelessness led someone to make the unthinkable decision to walk away from a sick little boy.

God calls His people to love and care for orphans, widows, and the sick and dying. Jagadish's plight, like so many other precious children, did not go unseen by their heavenly father who brought them to the Home of Hope. The hopelessness that threatened to overcome Jagadish was pushed back by the power of God's love.

Hope won for Jagadish and hope will continue to prevail. "Runners are the feet of the miracle that God is doing in India," reflected runner, Rich Cowman who had the chance to visit India and see the Home of Hope first hand.

In an unlikely partnership, runners are purposely choosing pain and suffering (52.4 miles in four weeks always results in some pain!) and through their sacrifice of love, children a half a world away are finding their pain lessened. Small steps of obedience are changing the world, one step at a time.

COMPELLED BY LOVE

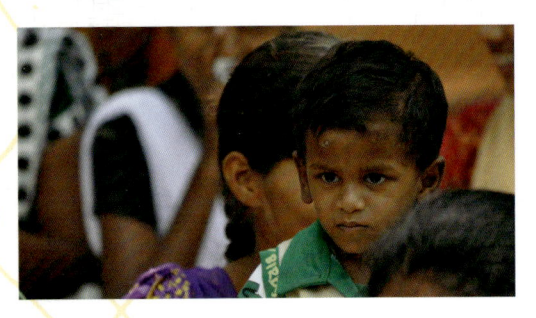

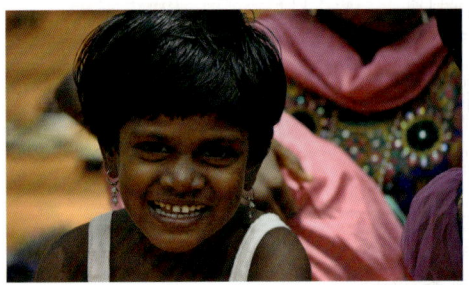

ANNA MORENO

Heaven's Gate Runner Anna Moreno wrote this song after a visit to the Home of Hope in India. As she was leaving, a little girl looked up at Anna and said, "Don't forget about me." These words haunted Anna and inspired the words to this song. To hear it, go to www.run4heavensgate.org.

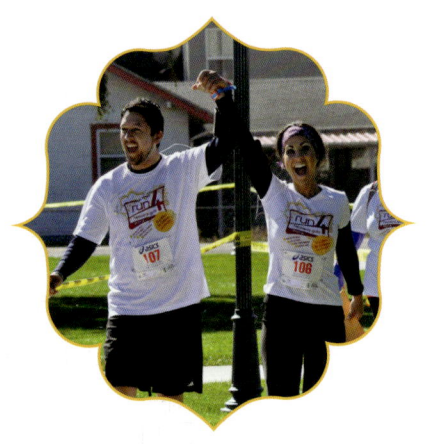

Anna and husband, Pablo

DON'T FORGET ABOUT ME

Brown eyes filled with tears
Lips that say don't forget about me
Markings on my skin,
Though they fade
Don't forget about me
I'll think of you
I won't forget about you
When lightning flashes down
With floods of rain
Don't forget about me
Remember God is love
He's your sunshine
As the days grow gray
Think of me I won't forget about you

Sweet child run with all you have
Go shine your light for all to see
And believe you're meant to change the world
And don't give up
'Cause hope never runs out
Think of me, I won't forget about you

Oh oh dry your eyes, love is by your side
Oh oh dry your eyes, love is by your side

Anna Moreno

COMPELLED BY LOVE

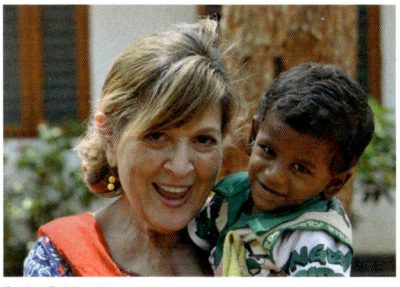

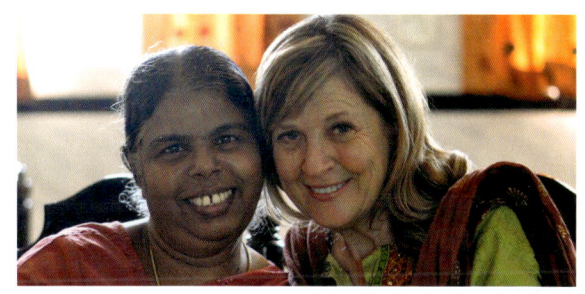

Cathy Caldwell

Cathy with Victoria, Pastor Guna's wife

CATHY CALDWELL

Choosing to participate in the Run 4 Heaven's Gate season held a more personal meaning for Cathy Caldwell than maybe any other runner. Cathy has been a key part of all of the work being done in India from the time it was only a prayer. Together with her husband Bob, she has been to India over 50 times. "I ran because I love India, and our children and family there. Participating in the Run 4 Heaven's Gate is one way we can convey our love to our children in India. They need to know that we are family, even though a world away, we pray for them, we love them, and will do what ever we can for them, we are compelled by love."

Cathy isn't a runner or distance walker on her own, "I know we can do things that we never imagined when we step out in faith and take hold of God's hand." Cathy experienced this as she battled through foot pain during training and completing each race.

Traveling to India twice a year for over 25 years has given Cathy a personal and first hand understanding of the realities of life for children and families there. "I have discovered the heart of God in a way I have never known before as I have watched our brothers and sisters in India reach out to help those who are destitute and alone, suffering from the deadly disease of AIDS. I have seen the deeply intense love and passion that God has for those who have no helper, and the transforming beauty that occurs when each precious life has been touched by His love. It is this same love of God found in Christ Jesus that compels those who do the Heaven's Gate runs. It is a love that has counted the cost, and there is no cost too great to keep them from doing what they can to help make a difference for children and families in such great need."

"This is beautiful; this is God's heart."

COMPELLED BY LOVE

Dear Run 4 Heaven's Gate Team,

Greetings and best wishes from Calvary Chapel Trust, Bangalore. Because many participants may never, ever see these children, the HIV children under the care and protection of Calvary Chapel Trust, we would like to offer some insights regarding our child care intervention.

Statistics show that children infected with HIV from birth do not tend to live beyond 14 or 15 years. What we

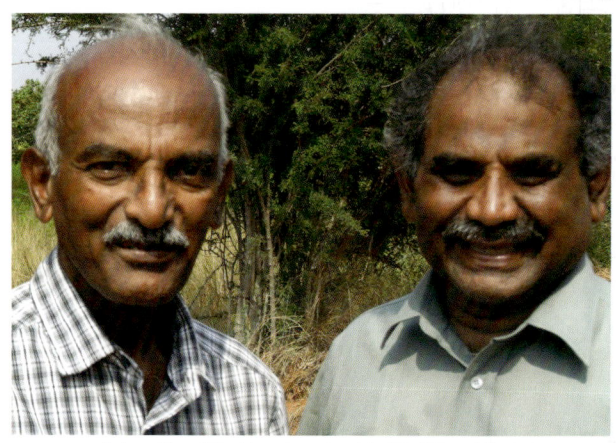

Calvary Chapel Trust board member John Wycliffe and Guna

have found is that with proper care and medication, their life span is being extended to beyond 22 years. HIV is a dreaded disease all over the world, yet here in India, it is wrapped in secrecy. This is because of the fear of being ostracized from family and community. When the children living in our Homes of Hope die an early death, most die as Christians. Many have left this world with Jesus on their lips.

Dying and un-reached children are plenty on the streets of India. Many are abandoned and left for dead. It is our desire to help more children. Your efforts are helping us to do this. Currently, we are only making a small impact compared to the need.

Run 4 Heaven's Gate team members, your burden is a noble one. Please remember, Jesus said, "Whatever you did for one of the least of these brothers of mine, you did for me" (Mathew 25:40). Just be re-assured that your cause will bring light to many and will be pleasant in the sight of God.

Please accept our best wishes for your event. God bless.

Yours in Christ,

Pastor Lamech Gunasekaran
Calvary Chapel Trust, Bangalore

COMPELLED BY LOVE

HOW YOU CAN SUPPORT SEND HOPE AND RUN 4 HEAVEN'S GATE

- Sign up to run 52.4 miles of love. (www.run4heavensgate.org/register)
- Start a Run 4 Heaven's Gate Team in your area. It only takes one person to get a team started. (And we will help you!)
- Support a runner. (www.run4heavensgate.org/sponsor)
- Sponsor a child. (Ask others to sponsor a child too!) (http://sponsor.sendhopenow.org/how-you-can-help/all-children)
- Pray for the children and caretakers in India.
- Host a bake sale or fundraiser for the kids in India.
- Follow Send Hope and Run 4 Heaven's Gate on Facebook and Instagram.
- Pray for a Run 4 Heaven's Gate Runner.
- Attend a race and encourage the runners, host a water station, donate to the cause, or share treats at the finish lines.
- Spread the word. Tell the story. Use your passion to help children!

FOR MORE INFORMATION ABOUT SEND HOPE AND RUN 4 HEAVEN'S GATE AND TO SEE WHAT IS NEW, VISIT US AT: RUN4HEAVENSGATE.ORG AND SENDHOPENOW.ORG

EMAIL: DOTTIE@RUN4HEAVENSGATE.ORG

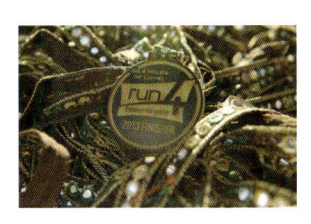

"I am only one, still I am one, I cannot do everything, but still I can do something. I will not refuse to do something I can do." – Helen Keller

COMPELLED BY LOVE

ACKNOWLEDGMENTS

This book has been a labor of love and partnership!

Our thanks to:

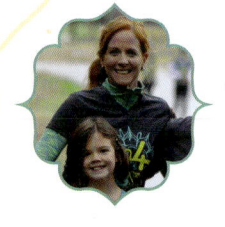

Dottie Bledsoe
Runner, Leader, Encourager.
Thanks for following
God's prompting!

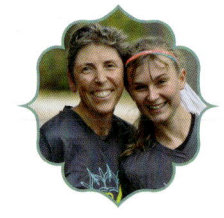

Maryanna Young
Runner, Publisher, Visionary.
Without you, this project
wouldn't have happened.

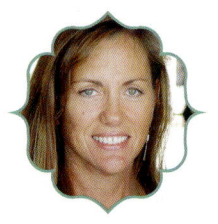

Lauren Phillips
Runner/Walker, Wise
Woman, Prayer Warrior.
We couldn't have done this
without your passion for
the children.

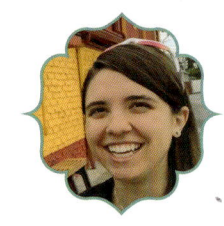

Hannah Cross
Runner (rookie season),
Editor, Project Manager.
Your eye for detail and
knowledge about serving
the poor added greatly
to this book.

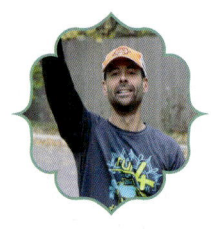

Doug McFerrin
Runner, Graphic Designer.
We appreciate your gift
of creativity.

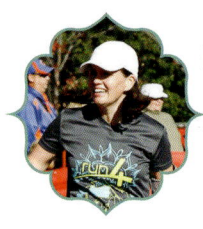

Amy Hoppock
Runner, Writer. The countless
hours you pored into this
project that flow from your
heart and passion for
serving these children has
blessed many.